AF880438

BUILDING NEW NURSING ORGANIZATIONS

Visions and Realities

Cathleen Krueger Wilson, PhD, RN
Senior Partner
Specialty Applications
Scottsdale, Arizona

AN ASPEN PUBLICATION®
Aspen Publishers, Inc.
Gaithersburg, Maryland
1992

Library of Congress Cataloging-in-Publication Data

Wilson, Cathleen Krueger.
Building new nursing organizations : visions and realities /
Cathleen Krueger Wilson.
p. cm.

Includes bibliographical references and index.
ISBN: 0-8342-0307-3
1. Nursing — Planning. I. Title.
[DNLM: 1. Nursing — organization & administration. 2. Nursing —
trends. WY 105 W747b]
RT89.W55 1992
362.1'73'068 — dc20
DNLM/DLC
for Library of Congress

Copyright © 1992 by Aspen Publishers, Inc.
All rights reserved.

Aspen Publishers, Inc., grants permission for photocopying for personal or internal use. This consent does not extend to other kinds of copying, such as copying for general distribution, for advertising or promotional purposes, for creating new collective works, or for resale. For information, address Aspen Publishers, Inc., 200 Orchard Ridge Drive, Gaithersburg, Maryland 20878.

Editorial Services: Ruth Bloom

Library of Congress Catalog Card Number: 91-22412
ISBN: 0-8342-0307-3

Printed in the United States of America

1 2 3 4 5

This book is dedicated to Carolyn, Bonnie, Julie, Wendy, and Maureen, nurses who taught me the true meaning of commitment.

Table of Contents

Contributors

Rhonda M. Anderson, MPA, CNAA
Senior Administrator
Good Samaritan Regional Medical Center
Phoenix, Arizona

Carol Hatler, BS, RN
Director of Administrative Services
Arizona Nurses Association
Tempe, Arizona

Kathy Malloch, MBA, RN
Clinical Nursing Administrator
Maryvale Samaritan Medical Center
Phoenix, Arizona

Doris Milton, PhD, RN
Director of Nursing Research
Maryvale Samaritan Medical Center
Phoenix, Arizona

Foreword

Everything is changing. The world is undergoing major transformation. From economics to political systems, whole societies are being reconfigured to reflect new realities and the death of old ideologies.

It is within this context that health care currently exists. In the United States, the promises of health care have not entirely been fulfilled. The relationship between the costs and the outcomes of health care has been poorly defined and the resultant impact on society has been dramatic. A heavily dominating medical model that looks at health care on an illness continuum has been inadequate to truly produce a healthier nation. Access to health care has been radically and negatively affected for a growing segment of the American population. Even for those who can afford to pay, the cost is accelerating while the benefit is depreciating. Clearly, newer approaches and models of health care delivery are essential if an adequate system of health service is to be provided in the United States.

The health care system is hungry for what nursing has to offer. Rather than having been illness focused, nursing is concerned about the continuum of healthy living and the services necessary to maintain and obtain health and healing. This concern goes beyond cure. The life continuum approach focuses on health as a process not as an event and thus provides for a broader context for the provision of services. These approaches to health care are exactly what the system needs. The challenge for nurses is to construct approaches within a reality that evidences viability in services, cost effectiveness, and defined and measurable outcomes. Newer models of delivery must be defined and developed in ways where their efficacy is evident and their impact is clear to payers, providers, and consumers of health care.

Furthermore, the circumstances of the times must be incorporated into the strategy of organizational and service transformation. As we move out of the Industrial Age into the Socio-Technical Age, nurses will have to become comfortable with high levels of organizational "noise," uncertainty, and constant and universal change. The old dependence on routines and stability in the work place is simply no longer an authentic circumstance. In transformational times such as our current era, people must learn to "journey" with the understanding that they may never fully arrive, instead of simply beginning the next phase of the voyage to an outcome that may not become clear for a long time. This kind of journeying may mean living more comfortably with adjustment, accommodation, dialogue, negotiation, and compromise. Relationships become vital. Therefore, collaboration, integration, and group process become more vital to the success of any venture.

This book deals effectively with all of these issues. Indeed, it creates a model for organizational change and identifies the major strategies that assist the change agents in making effective change in organizations. Furthermore, it describes approaches that best exemplify appropriate ways of dealing with the times and creating effective organizations in a time of great change. Using the information in this text, the reader will be well guided in the process of building new structures and models for service delivery. In addition to affecting the appropriate process of change, the author enumerates how to teach people to change and strategies for leading change.

It is my hope that *Building New Nursing Organizations: Visions and Realities* will be the first of many that clearly and effectively articulate the requisites of creativity and innovation as applied to the changing places where nurses practice their profession. Dealing with change as a living experience and structuring the requisite responses are vital to garnering success in delivering nursing services today and tomorrow.

This book provides both the insights and the tools necessary to that mission.

Tim Porter-O'Grady, EdD, RN, CS, CNAA
President
Tim Porter-O'Grady, Incorporated
Atlanta, Georgia

Preface

This book was developed as the result of many conversations with nurses across the country who are struggling with the implementation of new visions for nursing in the professional work place. As one of those nurses, I was struck by the lack of documentation of the real world challenges accompanying the introduction of a new order of things in nursing. Anyone who has introduced change has learned from their successes and their mistakes. However, the mistakes are rarely reported in the literature! It is my heartfelt hope that this work partially fills this gap.

In addition, the transformation of nursing work is an incredibly political activity. In my experience, this characteristic of change is one of the most difficult for nurses to discuss, except behind closed doors. Consequently, dealing with some of the interpersonal issues of change can be quite isolating at times. It is hoped that readers will find both validation of their observations, as well as several practical strategies for addressing the politics of restructuring.

The first five chapters describe the steps in the successful implementation of new nursing structures. Project management principles, change theory, leadership concepts, and organizational theory are woven together in order to provide a conceptual basis for implementation activities. The remaining chapters are a collection of actual restructuring projects that are representative of the changes currently underway in many nursing organizations. The authors have worked diligently to outline not only their original vision of a new nursing structure but the challenges and obstacles associated with their implementation.

Although not stated, a major assumption in this book is that nursing organizations commonly function within the context of a larger health care organization. Readers are encouraged to apply those key organizational concepts to the larger organization, if this fits their present situation.

This book is the end-product of the love, friendship, and colleagueship of many individuals, many who are pioneers. My husband, Ward, and my son, Ryan, remained steadfast in their support and loyalty which helped me to stick with the project. The pioneering nurses of Scottsdale Memorial Hospital-Osborn allowed me to participate with them in the development of a new participative structure. Many of them put their hearts and souls into the change, and their honesty taught me much about the personal experience of change. Ann Lewis and David Gyongyous, by engaging in vigorous debate and discussion about the nature of restructuring activities, helped me to more clearly formulate my thoughts. Their support and friendship are cherished. Without the thorough work and understanding of Betty Yokshas, the manuscript would never have been typed. Finally, this book would never have been conceived without the encouragement of Tim Porter O'Grady, whose steadfast commitment to a new nursing vision has been a continual source of inspiration to me.

Cathleen Krueger Wilson

CHAPTER 1

Transforming Our Nursing Future

"There is nothing more difficult to take in hand, more perilous to conduct or more uncertain in its success than to take the lead in the introduction of a new order of things."

—*Machiavelli, 1592*

There is no doubt that our nursing organizations need to change. Our present organizational structures and delivery systems, in most instances, lack the sophistication to keep pace with demands for greater flexibility, sensitivity to consumer demands, cost-effectiveness, and improved quality of care.

The American health care system is in a shambles, with patient care becoming increasingly impersonal and fragmented. Demands for change are coming from all directions. Nurses are the heart of the system and have the unique opportunity to participate in the transformation of health care. Will we be a part of the problem or will we lead the way to solution? Which will you choose? Here are some startling trends which suggest that we must choose to transform our nursing structures:

- Consumers continue to have concerns about the cost and the quality of health care. Two-thirds of Indiana residents support some form of national health care, even if it means raising taxes.[1]
- Nurse executives are increasingly required to minimize the negative effects of cost-control quality care required.
- Many of the nation's hospitals are in financial trouble. Maine's 42 acute care and specialty hospitals had operating losses in 1989 which were four times greater than losses in the previous year.[2]

Iowa hospitals averaged a negative 2.6% operating margin in 1989.[3]

- Payers, policy-makers, and providers are forced to address rationing and access to health care as the number of uninsured or inadequately insured Americans increases rapidly. There are an estimated 37 million uninsured persons in the United States today. Forty-six percent are full-time workers and their families who do indeed utilize health care services.[4]
- The financial crisis facing hospitals has resulted in the loss of needed services in many areas across the country. A strip along a highway in Texas is called the "dead zone" because hospital closures have resulted in no hospitals being open for hundreds of miles.[5]
- A huge industry has developed to monitor health care costs and force changes in service delivery. Pressures to reduce costs are negatively influencing care, in some instances. Patients are being discharged while still requiring more care for the episode for which they had been admitted, while readmissions are on the rise.
- New areas of hospital liability include patient falls and other complications due to understaffing, and adverse side effects from new technology[6] when competition for patients is put ahead of risk management.
- Health care is moving to the out-patient setting. Independent recovery care centers are springing up and attracting the more profitable patients from the acute care setting—at 25% to 30% lower costs.[7]
- Length of stay is dropping, acuity is rising, and fewer nursing hours are being used to care for patients.[8] This trend is putting extraordinary demands upon nursing delivery systems.
- The recruitment and retention of qualified nurses remains an issue. Only 50% of nurses work in hospitals 12 years after graduation, and of those who do, over 1/3 work in nonstaff positions.[9]
- Medicare cuts totalled $43 billion dollars in the FY 1991 budget approved by Congress. These cuts will influence the services made available to the increasing number of elderly patients using health care services in the United States.[10]

- Hospitals are not the secure employers they once were. Layoffs, small raises, and reduced benefits have combined with chaotic environments to create an atmosphere of crisis. Traditional unions are targeting health care organization, as uncertainty and disgruntlement are on the rise.

DEFINING RESTRUCTURING

In every arena, health care organizations are facing intense and competing demands for quality care and a quality work place. Successful nursing organizations are thriving in the face of such adversity, by taking the opportunity to build both new organizational structures and to improve management practices.

The term "restructuring" is used widely in nursing circles to describe many kinds of change. For the purposes of this book, restructuring refers to those major change initiatives that might include: the reduction of costs by being leaner, the alteration of nursing practices to gain greater focus, the discontinuation of those activities unrelated to core competencies and the creation of new organizational structures which permit participation, stimulate innovation and flex in response to competing demands.[11]

The restructuring of a nursing organization is clearly a major change initiative. The successful design of new nursing structures will depend upon the effectiveness of project planning, management, and evaluation. Later chapters examine the issues related to each stage of project management, as described in Figure 1–1.

Project conception is initiated when there begins to be awareness about the limitations of a particular nursing structure. At this stage, the nursing organization moves towards problem definition through the initial assessments of strengths and weaknesses. Faltering nursing structures are examined in order to better understand the gap between how the structure is actually performing and how it needs to perform in order to meet current demands. Symptoms of poor performance are noted, along with past attempts to remedy the situation. The needs of various users, the readiness of the organization for change, the identification of potential solutions, and the delineation of general goals for the change project are also examined in great detail. This stage culminates with the production of a realistic assessment of nursing structure perfor-

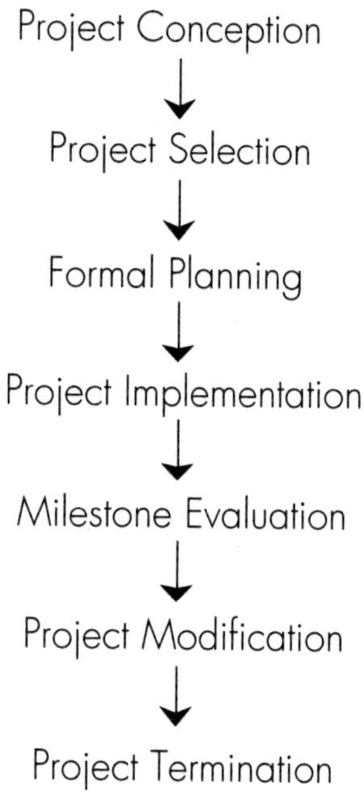

Figure 1-1 Stages of a Nursing Restructuring Project. *Source:* Information from *Managing Projects in Organizations* by J.D. Frame, pp. 103–110, Jossey-Bass Publishers, © 1987.

---

mance, organizational strengths and weaknesses, and a list of potential solutions.[12]

Next, the organization enters into the project selection stage. At this junction in the project cycle, choices must be made among the potential solutions, the needs of multiple users of the nursing structure, and the value of a new structure to the whole organization. If these differing requirements can be linked together in a meaningful way, then a decision to change can be finalized.[13]

Formal planning follows the decision to change. Identification of project time lines and outcomes, selection of a project team, delineation of implementation strategies, and selection of an evaluation methodology are the key activities encompassed in this stage of the project cycle.

Project implementation includes those activities for initiating a change, including re-education strategies, communication methods, and controlling functions.

Milestone evaluation and project modification phases follow implementation and include the pilot evaluation and ongoing evaluations of a change, which are then used to modify the project design, if such alteration is warranted. The project is terminated with a final evaluation of the overall change.

Some restructuring projects are aimed at increasing managers' access to professional knowledge and empowering staff participation in decisions. These initiatives hope to minimize the negative effects of competing demands for cost-effectiveness and quality, while also retaining professional nurses. Other restructuring projects are designed to streamline inefficient management structures and nursing roles. The goals of such projects may include cost reduction and provision of the supports necessary for quality nursing care, while increasing flexibility and responsiveness to patient care needs in an ever-changing environment. In the former, the organizational structure is the focus of the project while in the latter the redesign of a delivery system is the heart of the change project.

RESTRUCTURING THE DIVISION OF LABOR

The restructuring of an organization can be defined as a radical departure from the manner in which an organization divides its labor into distinct tasks as well as a change in the activities used to coordinate the tasks. The design of a nursing organization will reflect the unique pattern of those significant relationships that influence planning, communication, objective setting, controlling, and evaluation activities. Also, several interpersonal factors, critical to successful change, are influenced by organizational structure. These include leadership styles, commitment to the organization, and satisfaction with nursing work. At the same time, the structure of an organization is extremely sensitive to certain characteristics of the organization itself. The influence of organizational age, size, technology, and environment are important features to examine when considering a change in structure.[14]

Restructuring the division of labor occurs whenever tasks are rearranged in order to improve the chance of meeting a goal or to meet the demands of a new goal. In such a change, job descriptions are revised, along with reassignment of responsibility, new delegations of authority, and new guidelines for the manner in which the structure is linked to the organizational mission.

In fact, the division of labor will have a significant influence on individual performance. In the successful management of change, leaders will recognize that the obstacles presented may not only be due to individual behaviors but also may be due to obstacles created by the organizational structure itself.

In new age nursing organizations, the division of labor is being altered in order to 1) reduce emphasis upon hierarchy for effectiveness 2) nurture autonomy and accountability for greater quality care 3) replace rules in favor of professional nursing judgement, and 4) to increase utilization of a precious resource. In this book, the implementation of shared governance models and the implementation of product line management in a rehabilitation hospital are offered as real world examples of restructuring projects that significantly alter the division of labor in nursing organizations.

Nursing leaders must carefully approach the initiation of new organizational structures. If the change process does not include a careful analysis of the present structure and of organizational characteristics, then the new nursing structure will not be integrated into the whole health care organization, resulting in poor performance and disharmony.

CHANGING THE NURSING DELIVERY SYSTEM

Many nursing organizations are today engaged in the purposeful redesign of nursing work. Multiple needs are driving these changes, including the need to fill nursing vacancies, reduce costs for service delivery, maximize efficiency, reduce turnover and/or dissatisfaction, and maintain or maximize quality. This type of change project is challenging because of the requirement to sort the needs of multiple users.[15]

What needs fixing? Many nurses today are struggling to deliver care under archaic delivery systems which, in fact, hamper their efforts. For example, nursing work is not assigned by task difficulty and skill level, to the frustration of both patient and nurse. Nurses are simply not matched to patient needs. Patient assignments do not take into account the significant affective and cognitive requirements of care. Consequently, nursing practice is largely comprised of those activities that require psychomotor skills. Yet, the increase in acuity and complexity of care requires delivery systems that allow nurses time to think. Finally, shortages and cutbacks have resulted in the addition of significant administrative or non-nursing work to the nursing workload.[16] The tendency to continue to add responsibilities to the nursing role, in the face of shortages and cutbacks, burdens the nurse so much that nursing care and the nurse's satisfaction with the care delivered truly suffers.

In delivery system redesign, project concept definition must begin with the delineation of the role of the nurse, extending outward to levels of extenders and expanded roles. Armed with a clear definition, nursing leaders will be able to assure that delivery system changes will not only enhance the practice of professional nursing but also assure the quality of care in a cost-effective manner. In the chapters to follow, two cases are offered as examples of delivery system design: the implementation and evaluation of differentiated practice model and the implementation of evaluation strategies when delivery systems are being redesigned at multiple sites.

PROJECT CONCEPTION

Clearly both opportunity and risk are inherent in the implementation of new nursing structures. How does one design and implement a plan which will optimize the opportunities yet minimize the risk? Through informal preplanning and assessment, the nursing leader can identify the demands driving the need for change, prioritize the needs of multiple users, determine if a change is really warranted, examine the ability of the organization to facilitate support or obstruct the change, and evaluate the nursing culture's acceptance of innovations.

Identifying and Prioritizing Needs

Where is the need for change coming from? Is the need for change being driven by external forces, as in a crisis, or from a purposeful strategic initiative of the nursing department? When change is perceived as being forced upon an organization, the preplanning stage must carefully identify areas of potential resistance so that implementation will be accompanied by the persuasion and the education of resistors.

What are the needs that are being expressed? The need for shared governance may arise from an identified lack of organizational commitment, the existence of unclear nursing roles, a need to balance participation and direction, a demand to define nursing within the organization, a search for increased opportunities for growth, or a requirement to improve information and communication.

Are the needs being expressed the real needs for change? For example, nursing managers may express a need to change the nursing delivery system because of an increase in the number of vacant positions. Is this the real need? Perhaps the real need is to change the delivery system so that nursing work is satisfactory and results in increased recruitment and retention. The accuracy of need definition will be improved by reading literature which describes the problems, by reviewing the solutions attempted by similar organizations, and by talking to as many people affected by the need as is necessary.[17]

Whose needs will be met by the implementation of a new nursing structure? The demand for change may be the culmination of multiple needs. Administrators are looking for cost-effectiveness or are perhaps working towards the next promotion. Nursing leaders may want to strengthen nursing as well as their position in the organization. Clinical nurse specialists may want to improve the state of the art in their specialty and staff nurses may want to have more control over their practice.

How can these multiple and diverse needs be addressed? Frame (1987) suggests that a "need hierarchy" be developed in order to clarify, list, and prioritize competing needs for change. This hierarchy is essentially a schematic drawing of the needs to be addressed by a particular project and the level of priority assigned to each need. Figure 1-2 is an example of a needs hierarchy for the implementation of a shared governance model.

Figure 1-2 describes an overall need to improve the performance of the nursing department. In this hypothetical nursing department, there are a number of vacant nursing positions, coupled with an increasing number of nurses moving into pool positions. The nursing work environment operates on crisis management. Shared governance is being considered as a partial solution to these problems.

The next level of specific needs that could be met by moving to a shared governance model includes: the reduction of the number of vacancies and turnover, improved nursing productivity, and increased commitment and job security. Each of these needs must be identified in order of priority at this level. Which is the most important? The nature of the shared governance model eventually selected for implementation is dependent upon such prioritization.

A third level of needs is found under each of the three major identified needs at level 2. For example, improved productivity is sure to occur when the education function is transformed so that both nursing and management education needs are met. As managers are freed from

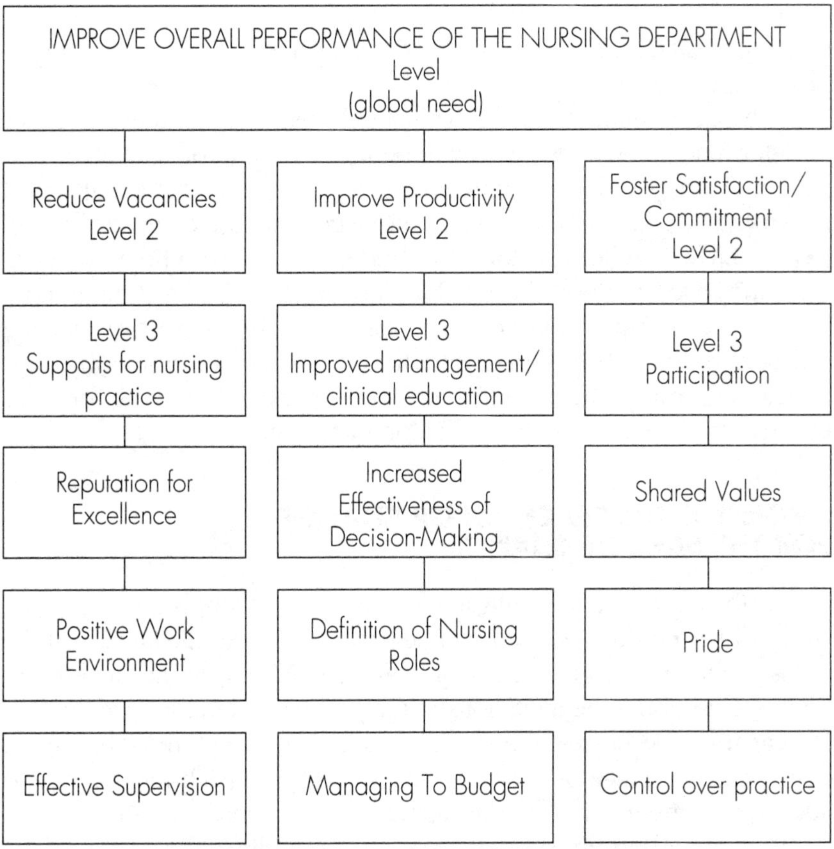

Figure 1-2 A Needs Hierarchy for Shared Governance Model Implementation

clinical decisions and those at the bedside gain control of nursing clinical decisions, the efficiency of decision making across the organization will see improvement. Finally, as nursing practice moves into the hands of practitioners, nursing roles will be streamlined and improved to meet the requirements for quality care. Once again, at this level, the priorities need to be determined. Which of the needs identified here are the most emergent? This level prioritization will determine the order in which nursing department functions are transformed to a shared governance process.

Although this needs hierarchy stops at level three, it can and should be extended as part of the formal planning process so that communication about priorities for the change is clear, milestones are accurately identified, and evaluation strategies are directed to the appropriate outcomes.[18]

The development of a needs hierarchy enables the nursing leader to determine just whose needs will be met by the implementation of a new structure. Examining Figure 1-2 again, it appears that a major goal is to increase commitment and job satisfaction. Whose commitment and job satisfaction? Who will participate and share values? Who will experience increased pride in the nursing department? Who will have more control over nursing practice? Who will have less control over nursing practice? By completely specifying all of the needs to be met by a restructuring project, the nursing leader can lay the groundwork for more effective planning and implementation of change.

AVOIDING THE QUICK FIX OR CHANGE FOR THE SAKE OF CHANGE

Is the new structure really a new approach or simply a repackaging of the old, accompanied by the same flaws as prior to the change? If the focus of the change is the nursing delivery system, does accurate information exist about the limitations of the present system? For example, is it clear how the nurses, the staffing levels, and the work environment combine to enhance or obstruct the present system?[19] If the answers to such questions are not readily apparent, one must be careful about rushing into a delivery system change without eliminating some of the limitations of the present system. Similarly, a specialty program may be failing for a variety of reasons including poor decisions from prior management, inaccurate marketing information, a shift in patient population, or poor supervision. A change to product line management will carry all of these inadequacies along with it, dooming the project to certain failure.

It is human nature to be dazzled by the promise of the new. However, if flaws in current operations are not identified early on, project failure and lost opportunities for efficiency and quality are sure to follow. The prospect of negative outcomes can be minimized by taking the time to examine the status quo prior to selecting a certain direction.

Nursing organizations and the people who work in them seem particularly vulnerable to change for the sake of change. This characteristic of some organizations has been referred to as "entrepreneurialism run rampant over sound management principles."[20] Those experiencing a need for change may be so caught up in the religiouslike fervor of an identified solution that significant problems will be overlooked. For example, although every nursing department in town is implementing case management, it will be wiser to wait to change until the problem has been clearly defined. In this way the solution selected is more likely to meet identified needs for a particular organization.

IDENTIFYING ORGANIZATIONAL RESOURCES

In the preplanning phase, the nursing leader is challenged to put together a preliminary list of what the project would require in terms of resources, should it be implemented. In particular, it is important to ascertain if there is a gap between the project concept and the real world. Final project selection is based upon this critical assessment.[21] Pertinent questions include:

- Will there be enough time, enough knowledge, and enough staff to implement the new structure?
- Is the organization willing to change policies, including personnel policies, in order to meet the requirements of the new nursing performance?
- Is the nursing control system adequate to both facilitate evaluation and monitor performance?
- Does the management philosophy of the health care organization fit with the restructuring being proposed?
- If management philosophies are different, can differences be reconciled?

Without adequate resources over the long term, a restructuring project will fail. People, time, and knowledge needs must be identified so that formal planning includes adjustments for the loss and the replacement of these critical factors. Genuine change will be difficult to achieve if the organizational environment, particularly policies and procedures, remains unchanged. Individuals and groups vary in their readiness for change and change always includes unanticipated events that at times require rapid detection and intervention.

An effective management control system is critical for accurate monitoring and evaluation during implementation. How is the nursing department divided into areas of accountability and how is performance monitored? Is there a major difference in management philosophies and if there is, what processes will be used to address conflicts? The management environment will influence the political support for the change as well as those involved in leading it. The final selection of a restructuring project must be, in part, based upon the degree of congruence between the organization and the new nursing structure.

PREDICTING COORDINATION PROBLEMS

The coordination processes of an organization are most sensitive to errors in design. Consequently, early thinking about the project must consider how the coordination of patient care may be altered during and after the implementation of new nursing structures. What coordination practices exist in the current environment? How will these be influenced during the implementation of a change? What can be done to minimize negative effects? Will the proposed change strengthen the coordination of patient care? How?

For example, some product line management models will significantly alter coordination responsibilities assigned to the traditional head nurse role. How will these coordination functions be identified and reassigned? How will coordination shifts be monitored for effectiveness during implementation? Clearly, coordination issues must be considered in the project conception phase, so that the selected design meets coordination requirements. Differences in coordination processes in simple and complex organizations are highlighted in Figure 1-3.

For example, in a small home health nursing agency, mutual adjustment or coordination through staff cooperation is common. If the

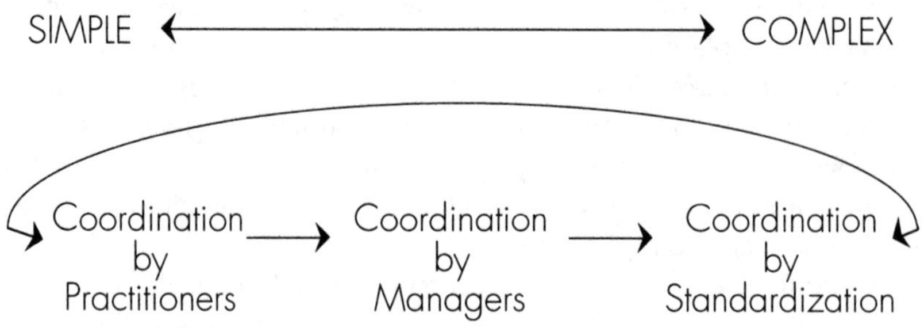

Figure 1-3 Coordination Issues and Organizational Complexity

agency grew significantly in size, patient care would suffer because of competing demands for coordination. Managers would be added to ease the burden of coordination from the staff group.[22] If the agency took on more services and grew in complexity as in the case of the acute care hospital, coordination would also be achieved through standardization of some work processes.

In highly specialized services, the outcome of the care is often standardized, leaving the practitioner the choice of processes used to deliver the care. At the same time, the more specialized a service is, the more likely a supervisor will not be the most knowledgeable about the actual work. Thus, consideration must be given to placing some of the coordination of the care into the hands of the practitioner.[23]

In most organizations, there is usually a mix of coordination practices. As an organization increases in size and complexity, standardization of work, management processes, and the authority of practitioners become predominant controlling processes.[24]

ANTICIPATING INTEGRATION NEEDS

New nursing structures rearrange nursing functions in order to improve the chances of meeting an old goal or in order to meet the demands of a new goal. New differentiations of nursing work are evidenced in revisions of job descriptions, reassignments of responsibility, new delegations of authority for outcomes, new management structures, and new guidelines for the manner in which the nursing organizational structure is linked to the goals of the whole organization. When considering a restructuring proposal, the nursing leader can optimize success by assuring that there is an appropriate match between the new structure and certain environmental factors.[25]

The matching of nurses and nursing organization functions is no easy accomplishment. Success is contingent upon both the nature of the work and the needs of the nurses involved. In a complex hospital organization, any change in the organizational structure of the nursing department and the integration of such changes into the whole organization can be significantly compromised by certain characteristics of individuals and groups, as listed in Exhibit 1-1.

Differences in the characteristics of nurses most affected by the change and the amount of stereotyping across nursing groups will result

Exhibit 1-1 Integration Barriers

- Differences in nurses' preparation experience and skill level
- Differences in the goals/interests of nursing as compared to other departments
- Degree of reliance upon nursing ritual over patient outcome
- Amount of stereotyping across nursing groups
- Communication problems internal and external to the nursing department
- Priority given to nursing unit needs over the needs of the nursing department
- Number of differences between the new nursing structure and other departments

in varying levels of understanding and acceptance. Nurses vary considerably in educational preparation, experience, and degree of involvement in their work. To the extent that such differences are sharp between individuals and groups, implementation could be slowed dramatically.[26]

Divergent opinions may exist among individuals and groups regarding those behaviors that must remain and those that can be discarded, reflective or varying levels of reliance upon nursing ritual. The degree and number of different opinions will produce varying degrees of acceptance and commitment to the new structure.

The implementation of a new nursing organization structure may also be compromised by the degree of autonomy expressed by different units within the nursing department. Consequently, feedback about the effectiveness of the new structure and the commitment to making it work may be limited by the tendency of some nursing units or services to pay more attention to their own internal issues, rather than to fully participate in the change.[27]

Varying communication structures, both internal and external to the nursing department, can be problematic if individuals and groups receive information at differing times, in varying amounts, and with differences in accuracy. Differences in communication processes may result in unnecessary confusion and resultant coordination problems or, even worse, foster significant misperceptions about the change.

Finally, the integration of a new nursing organization into the whole health care organization can be slowed down by the degree of differences between the new nursing structure and the structures of other departments. Departments may vary from each other and from the nursing department in the goal orientation, communication structure, environmental focus, management authority structure, and time orientation.[28] Successful integration of new nursing organizational structures will be dependent upon the effectiveness of strategies designed to reduce conflict and create new opportunities for communication between nursing and other departments.

Integration issues will influence the selection of a new design and strategies for implementation. In particular, boundary spanning activities will be necessary to assure appropriate integration. The integration of new nursing structures is an important focus in project management and is discussed in greater detail in the chapters ahead.

EXAMINING THE NURSING ENVIRONMENT FOR OPENNESS TO CHANGE

How open is the nursing organization to change? Some organizations wait until a major crisis before reluctantly admitting a need for new structures. Other nursing organizations possess a culture committed to excellence. The degree of readiness and acceptance for change influences not only project selection but also implementation and monitoring strategies. If a nursing organization is perceived to be comfortable with change, when in reality it is not, the wrong project may be selected or the application of inadequate implementation strategies will obstruct goal achievement.

There are essentially eight characteristics of nursing organizations committed to excellence:[29]

1. a bias for action
2. exceptional care of the customer
3. constant innovation through autonomy and entrepreneurship
4. commitment and productivity through people
5. hands on, value driven leadership
6. sticking to the knitting
7. simple form and lean staff
8. simultaneous loose and tight properties

A bias for action is evidenced in a nursing organization by a culture which supports experimentation and informal problem solving. Communication flows from all directions, reflective of a networking organization whose central purpose is the provision of quality care. Problem solving is initiated by those most knowledgeable of the problem and potential solutions. Those who initiate problem solving most often also have the authority to implement solutions.[30]

In the implementation of new nursing structures, a nursing organization with a bias for action is more likely to be comfortable with the notion of change. It is also tolerant of implementation errors or design problems and encourages participation and risk-taking. In addition, any change is perceived from a futuristic perspective.[31] These attitudes and behaviors can stimulate excitement and increase the probability of success.

Excellent nursing organizations are committed to achieving quality nursing care. This focus is evidenced in the definitions of change projects. Definitions are always tied in some way to enhancing quality care. The nursing quality assurance programs of excellent nursing organizations are strong, providing effective resources for the monitoring and evaluation of restructuring projects.

Nurses working in excellent organizations view themselves and others as trustworthy and unique individuals who expect partnerships and who enjoy their work. This is a people-valuing culture. A people-valuing culture assists in the implementation of new nursing structures because of the ease with which collaboration occurs and because nurses will involve themselves in facilitating the successful implementation of new structures.[32] In addition, innovation and experimentation are rewarded in excellent nursing organizations, fostering the necessary problem solving associated with the implementation of new designs.

In excellent organizations, nursing work is clearly defined and limited to what nursing does best. This assures that the selection of a restructuring project will be based on similar standards. Also, changes in organizational structure will be limited to those features which enhance the provision of care.

Finally, an excellent organization knows when to tightly control a function and when to let it be more decentralized.[33] This knowledge is useful when implementing change because coordination and integration issues are controlled but creativity and experimentation are not limited.

RESTRUCTURING PROJECT DEMANDS AND THE NURSE LEADER

This book is written for those pioneering nurses who have the major responsibility for a restructuring initiative. Leading a major change can be exhilarating and rewarding work. However, the health care environment produces demands to improve productivity while scaling down expenses. These outcomes must be achieved while also maintaining quality in the midst of rapid change. Such demands have created a conflicting set of expectations for the leaders of major change in health care organizations.

Prior to making a commitment to implement a new nursing structure, nursing leaders are well advised to conduct a personal inventory of those resources that can be drawn upon to provide the steadfastness, perseverance, and strength necessary for effective leadership of change in these stressful times. Rosebeth Moss Kanter (1987) adeptly describes some of the stressors facing the leaders of changing organizations, particularly the existence of competing role demands.[34] Exhibit 1-2 contains a list of pertinent questions for the assessment of competing role demands.

Chances are, the answer to most of the questions in Exhibit 1-2 is yes. A careful sensitivity to the presence of these competing demands and the use of purposeful tactics devised to minimize their negative personal and organizational impact is critical to successful change. Without such sensitivity, the courage to take the next step, the strength to deal with obstacles and the sensitivity to the human experience of change will diminish the leadership so critically needed to guide an organization through a major restructuring process.

Some nursing leaders have developed support networks among those who are implementing similar changes (such as the now annual shared governance conference), in order to minimize the personal tolls of the change process and to learn from the experience of others. Both formal and informal support systems are necessary for success. The use of an outside consultant is also helpful, since the objectivity of this individual can lead to the validation of concerns, identification of obstacles, and applaud movement, no matter how small. Finally, the nursing leader must be able to set clear boundaries in order to stay centered and balanced in the midst of ambiguity.

To develop the organization of the future, we must have nursing leaders who have the resources to challenge the status quo, adventure

Exhibit 1-2 Assessing Leadership Role Demands

• Are you expected to think strategically and invest in the future, but keep the beds full, the staffing lean, and not spend too much on facilities improvement?	YES	NO
• Are you told to be entrepreneurial, innovative, and to take risks but not to make costly mistakes by failing?	YES	NO
• Do you expect yourself to continue to do everything you are doing even better: empower your nursing staff, conduct research, introduce innovation, meet the budget as well as to spend more time with your nursing staff?	YES	NO
• Are you required to know every detail related to the nursing organization but told to give more accountability to others?	YES	NO
• Do you find yourself passionately addicted to your vision of professional nursing and quality care, strongly committed to achieving these goals but struggling with flexibility, openness to new ideas, and having problems changing directions quickly?	YES	NO
• Do you throw yourself fully into entrepreneurial or intrapreneurial activity, regardless of the long hours it takes but expect yourself to stay fit and to raise terrific kids?	YES	NO

into unknown territory, and take risks. To take such risks is to go beyond the organizational injunction of "Don't fix what isn't broken" and act upon what is required to build nursing organizations for the future.

OUTCOMES OF SUCCESSFUL RESTRUCTURING

How does one really know if the change was a good one? A thoughtful, well-designed, effectively implemented and evaluated restructuring project will have certain outcomes, beyond those pertinent to the change itself:[35]

1. The structures which remain after restructuring will have added value to patient care activities.
2. Cost-cutting strategies are clearly aligned with improving delegation downward, creating a high commitment organization.

3. Redeployment is the hallmark of the change process, so that good people are reassigned to other parts of the system. This breeds trust, security, and commitment to the future.
4. Time is no longer spent on costly, labor intense services that detract from the provision of quality care. Nursing roles reflect only nursing work.
5. The change is seen as long term and one of continuous improvement to assure quality. Planning and evaluation activities, as well as the allocation of resources, evidence the long-term point of view.
6. There is a clearly identified match between the organization's mission and philosophy and the new structure. Hiring practices, socialization of new employees, rewards/incentives, and administrative decision making exemplify this connection.

QUESTIONS TO GUIDE PROJECT CONCEPTION

1. What specific problems will be addressed through the implementation of a new nursing structure?
   - organizational structure problem
   - delivery system problem
   - nursing role/performance problem
   - coordination problem
   - integration problem
2. What needs are being expressed? Is there consensus among the needs being expressed? Will a change in the nursing structure meet these demands?
3. How will needs be prioritized? Which needs will be left unaddressed?
   - professional nursing needs
   - physician needs
   - consumer needs
   - support department needs
   - manager needs
   - hospital administration needs

4. Is the targeted nursing structure performing as it was originally intended to perform? Where are the performance gaps and how are structure performance problems manifested?
   - How many and which types of individuals and groups are affected by the poor performance?
   - How severe is the performance problem of the targeted nursing structure?
   - Will the nursing structure need to be modified or replaced?
   - Is the problem experienced in the same manner across the nursing organization? If not, how are differences manifested?
5. Is the organization open and ready for change?
   - Adhoc task forces are commonly called upon to solve problems.
   - There is a positive questioning attitude.
   - Reward systems are tied to innovation and excellence.
   - Trust exists.
6. Have there been past attempts to remedy the situation?
   - Which groups or individuals were involved?
   - What solutions were attempted?
   - Did the intervention succeed or fail? Why?
7. Do the basic resources exist within the organization to support the introduction of change?
   - leadership
   - information systems
   - time and money
   - environment
8. Is the rationale for the change accurate and realistic?
   - change for change sake
   - knee jerk response or quick fix
   - thoughtful project conception

NOTES

1. Currents in finance. (1990). *Hospitals,* November 20, 16.
2. Ibid., p. 17.
3. Currents in finance. (1990). *Hospitals,* November 5, 16.

4. Department of Health Services. (1989). *A Profile of Uninsured Americans: Research Findings 1.* PHS 89–443, p. 12.
5. An interview with Carol McCarthy. (1990). *Hospitals,* September 5.
6. Holthaus, D. (1988). Changing times creates new liability hotspots. *Hospitals,* September, 58–61.
7. Outpatient planning: Still more art than science? (1990). *Hospitals,* December, 26–32.
8. Aiken, L. (1988). *The Nursing Shortage: Explanations and Potential Solutions.* Paper presented at the Executive Nursing Conference. October 1988, Philadelphia, PA.
9. Roberts, M., Minnick, A., Ginzberg, E., and Curran, C. (1989). *A Commonwealth Fund Paper: What To Do About The Nursing Shortage.* New York: Commonwealth Fund, pp. 11–12.
10. The top 10 developments in U.S. health care, 1990. (1990). *Hospitals,* December 20, 38–40.
11. Moss Kanter, R. (1989). *When Giants Learn to Dance.* New York: Simon and Schuster Publishers, p. 57.
12. Frame, J.D. (1987). *Managing Projects In Organizations.* San Francisco: Jossey-Bass Inc., Publishers, pp. 103–110.
13. Ibid., pp. 7–8.
14. Mintzberg, H. (1979). *The Structuring of Organization.* Englewood Cliffs, NJ: Prentice-Hall, Inc., pp. 1–17.
15. Frame, J.D. (1987), pp. 103–127.
16. Donald, M.K. (1988). The transformation of bedside nursing. *Aspen's Advisor for Nurse Executives,* 4(3), December, 3.
17. Frame, J.D. (1987), pp. 108–114.
18. Ibid., pp. 120–123.
19. Munson, F.C., Beckman, J.S., Clinton, J., Kever, C., and Sims, L.M. (1980). *Nursing Assignment Patterns User's Manual.* Ann Arbor: University of Michigan Press, pp. 1–31.
20. Herzlinger, R.E. (1989). The failed revolution in health care. *Harvard Business Review,* March–April, 95.
21. Frame, J.D. (1987), pp. 6–10.
22. Mintzberg, H.C. (1979), pp. 227–249.
23. Ibid., p. 371.
24. Ibid., pp. 230–231.
25. Lawrence, P. and Larsch, J. (1967). Differentiation and integration in complex organizations. *Administration Science Quarterly,* 12(2), June, 1–47.
26. Ibid., pp. 1–2.
27. Fink, S.L., Jenks, R.S., and Willits, R.D. (1983). *Designing and Managing Organizations.* Homewood, IL: Richard D. Irwin, Inc. Publishers, pp. 45–91.

28. Larsch, J.W. (1977). Introduction to structural design of organizations. In *Organizational Behavior and Industrial Psychology*. Kenneth N. Wexley and Gary A Yukl (Eds). New York: Oxford University Press, pp. 256–261.

29. Peters, T. and Waterman, R.H. (1982). *In Search of Excellence*. New York: Harper & Row Publishers.

30. Nesbitt, J. (1984). *Megatrends*. New York: Warner Books, pp. 211–229.

31. Kramer, M. and Schmolenberg, C. (1988). Magnet hospitals Part I: Institutions of excellence. *Journal of Nursing Administration,* 18(2), 13–34.

32. Miller, L.M. (1984). *The American Spirit. Visions of A New Corporate Structure.* New York: Warner Books, p. 40.

33. Moss, Kanter R. (1989), pp. 55–90.

34. Ibid., pp. 20–21.

35. Ibid., pp. 90–117.

CHAPTER 2

Selecting the Right Project

Once a problem has been clearly defined, a search begins for potential solutions. This begins the next step in the restructuring project cycle: project selection. At the end of this stage, either a particular nursing structure has been selected as a solution or a decision has been made not to change. The final decision should be based on an extensive organizational assessment, during which time the functional requirements of possible new structures are examined in relationship to available resources and organizational characteristics.[1] The criteria for final project selection include the following:

1. Organizational strengths are maximized.
2. Organizational weaknesses can be minimized during implementation.
3. Necessary resources are either available or can be easily obtained.
4. Motivations of individuals and key groups can be facilitated for successful change.
5. Leadership styles within the organization are appropriate to implementation needs.
6. Expertise in nursing management exists at each management level in the nursing organization.

Difficult choices must be made. No one structure will be able to meet the demands identified by multiple users during project conception. Some demands will be forsaken for others, according to priority. The importance of project selection activities cannot be overestimated. Sometimes the time necessary for adequate assessment of alternatives is cut short because of demands for expediency or because of a general lack of knowledge. Unfortunately, the ultimate outcome will be a new structure that eventually fails because of inadequate resources or unanticipated organizational obstacles. The project selected will be the one believed to do the best job in meeting prioritized needs while matching resource and structure requirements.[2] The quality of a new structure's performance is directly related to the time spent collecting and processing strategic information. Figure 2-1 illustrates this relationship.

What happens when project selection and design are inadequate? Consider the following scenarios:

Scenario #1 A nursing organization chooses to implement a shared governance model in order to improve the overall productivity of the nursing department. Little time is spent on project selection and design. A model is quickly selected, planned for, and implemented.

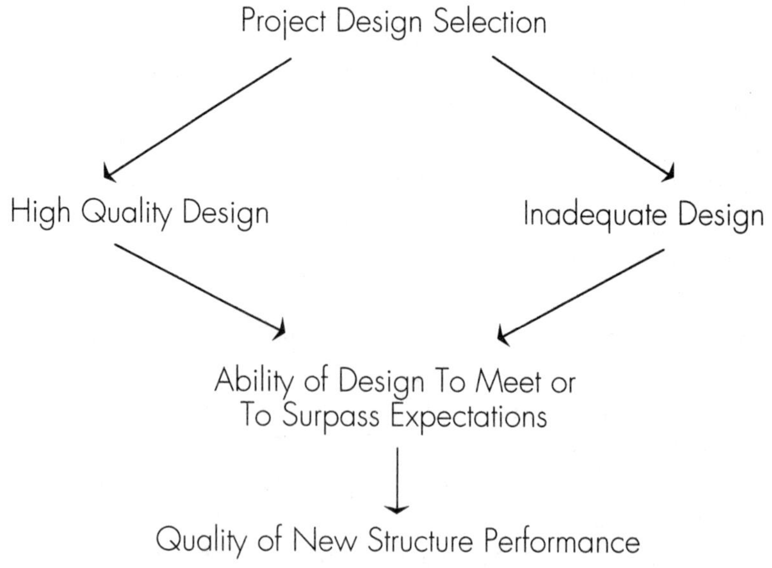

Figure 2-1 Project Design and Quality

Hospital administrators are confused about the new structure and have mixed feelings about it. Also, a lack of necessary nursing management skills is evident in the organization but not addressed in project selection. Consequently, planning and implementation strategies do not include education and/or persuasion of hospital administration. In addition, there is no planning for the acquisition of nursing management skills through recruitment and management development.

At the end of the second year of implementation, it is determined that shared governance is not working. The failure is partially due to nursing manager's fear of replacing clinical decision making in favor of increased management responsibilities, combined with a lack of support from hospital administration.

Scenario #2 Demands for increased cost-effectiveness and a reduction of staffing expenses resulted in a nursing organization deciding to change its nursing delivery system. The "quick fix" approach was the modus operandi in this organization. A limited literature review produced a model delivery system, which was quickly modified and adapted as the solution.

Inadequate project selection and design failed to identify the pre-existing nursing practice needs in the organization. There were no clinical specialists and relatively few baccalaureate nurses available to help in the definition of new nursing roles. The assignment of patients was largely based upon tasks rather than upon nurses' assessment and planning abilities or patient need. The result was a delivery system which introduced assistive personnel but utilized nurses and assistive personnel inappropriately. Nursing roles and functions, particularly the delegation functions, failed to meet professional and regulatory standards. These flaws resulted in abandonment of the project.

In the scenarios described, project selection did not match organizational requirements. The mismatch influenced planning and implementation. The new structure was erroneously rejected. The problem was not the concept itself, but an error in project design.

PROJECT SELECTION AND DESIGN IN PROFESSIONAL ORGANIZATIONS

Nursing organizations represent constellations of key activities believed to be necessary for quality patient care. They differ from one another with respect to age, size, services provided, technology, and environment. Differences are also found in the manner in which work is organized, the design and utility of planning and control systems, and the indirect staff support facilitating the major work of the organization.

Age

The older and larger a professional organization, the more formalized its behavior. As nursing organizations and the nurses who work in them age, work is repeated and simply becomes more predictable. The often heard phrase "we do it this way" becomes formalized in policy and procedures. Older organizations have limitations in energy, openness, and flexibility.[3] These features make the introduction of change a significant challenge for nursing leaders.

Simply put, aging organizations are not functioning as well as they used to in the past. Organizational systems may be inadequate to meet the demands of change. Employee support for the organization's goals may be superficial because of a simmering distrust. People are sensing that an ending is near.[4]

Yet, the successful introduction of new nursing structures requires that nurses with diverse viewpoints and trust levels put organizational goals ahead of self-interests. If this does not occur, then the interests of subsystems will erode the interests of the total organization. Self-interests are intensified when individuals perceive themselves at high risk to lose something of value to them. The realization of a common point of view among nurses with differing authority, varying power levels, individual professional identities, and various self-interests will occur if early on the change is introduced from a win–win perspective.

The project selected must be one that assures nurses there is a future and that the organization has a long-term commitment to them. This is particularly important in older organizations. Nurses will perceive commitment if such bread and butter issues as job security and benefits are guarded carefully during restructuring efforts. Also, if some good nurses lose their positions due to design requirements, then a place somewhere else in the organization must be found for them. In addition, nurses must be assured that increased productivity will not result in layoffs. The nursing culture must have trust as a key feature. Trust is developed in an organization where learning is nourished, people truly care for one another, and conflict is accepted as long as it is not driven by self-interest. Opportunities to discuss individual differences and to reveal concerns about change need to be planned. Otherwise, the implementation of a new nursing structure will erode commitment and permeate the environment with a win–lose perception of the change.

Project selection implies that some benefits will be forsaken in order to gain others. In the selection of a new structure, short-term losses must be identified. Once identified, then they can be linked to those long-term achievements that will be their replacement.[5] For example, in the implementation of shared governance, comfort with the predictable processes of clinical decision making will be temporarily replaced with ambiguity and confusion. In the long term, the loss of clear authority for clinical and management decision making will be replaced with strong nursing roles and decision-making processes that empower nurses and enhance quality care across the organization.

Older organizations present major barriers to the implementation of change. Whereas a growing organization ties risk-taking to success, the same behavior is studiously avoided in aging nursing organizations. Results exceed expectations in growing organizations, while in older organizations the reverse is true. During the implementation of new structures, the focus in aging organizations will be on "who is doing what" rather than upon planning and the rationale for the plan.[6]

In selecting a particular structure, nursing leaders must take into consideration the influence of age upon its successful implementation. The formal nature of aging organizations creates barriers to the necessary dialogue about the change and limits creativity. New liaison forums may need to be created in which nurses from across the organization can discuss a potential change and review relevant information. Clinical nurse specialists or other nurses in boundary-spanning roles can be used to move across the organization, discussing the change and collecting relevant information. Interestingly, in the implementation stage of a project, the formalization of aging organizations becomes a strength. It is then when rules for behavior will be important in order to minimize the role ambiguity accompanying a new order. Formalized communications during an implementation create an atmosphere of predictability in the midst of uncertainty.[7]

It is not easy to acknowledge that we may be a part of an aging organization and that our attitudes about nursing work and change may be significantly colored by this experience. However, a truthful assessment about the nursing organization's age and size and the identification of age-related barriers to a restructuring project will limit the possibility of disaster later in the change process. For example, a goal to move to a case management system may need to be delayed in an aging organization, preceded by a modification in the organizational structure that levels management layers and accompanying policies, and allows nurses to be entrepreneurs as well as employees.

Autonomy

Unlike other types of organizations, the standardization of work in professional organizations comes from external rather than internal sources. In particular, the standardization of nursing work is influenced by nursing education and by the promulgation of standards by professional associations.[8] Consequently, nurses are able to exert discretionary judgment when selecting nursing interventions. The direct supervision of nursing care is limited because it interferes with the autonomy of the nurse within the nurse–patient relationship. Not only do nurses have discretion in selecting which patient needs are to be responded to but also which organizational needs will be addressed.[9]

The autonomy of practitioners in professional organizations raises several challenges in the implementation of new nursing structures. The outcomes of nursing work are difficult to evaluate because of the autonomy of different nurses. The inability to directly supervise the provision of nursing care can result in the actions of incompetent or unconscientious nurses contributing to poor nursing structure performance.[10] The tendency may be to blame the design rather than recognize that systems for detecting substandard care are ineffective. In the project selection, care must be taken to examine proposed structures for performance monitoring needs. Systems that identify nurse performance issues may need to be developed early, so that implementation strategies are not impaired by poor performance.

Another issue related to autonomy is the difficulty in achieving consensus about *one* strategy for change. Professionals in organizations tend to reject any change that appears to be dividing professional work into standard pieces.[11] This is why the use of multiple pilot projects is particularly useful when implementing change in professional organizations. This design allows for the delineation of required structure functions, accompanied by specified allowances for differences. However, successful change through the use of multiple pilot units will be directly related to the clarity of definition for "required" versus "optional" design features.

Technology

Technology does not regulate the work of professional nurses. In fact, knowledge is the predominant technology within professional organizations. However, the sophistication of the technology needed for successful implementation will dramatically impact the performance of new nursing structures.

A lack of technical knowledge can limit nurses' understanding of a new structure's purpose and function. This misunderstanding will, in turn, lead to ineffective role behaviors during implementation. For example, a lack of manager expertise in delegating will produce inappropriate decision making during the implementation of shared governance. Similarly, the introduction of product line management may suffer greatly due to nurses' lack of knowledge about marketing. Knowledge needs relative to the new structure must be identified during project selection and design in order to avoid the emergence of inappropriate role behaviors later on. If knowledge needs are too numerous, a decision not to change until knowledge is advanced may be the best choice.

Because of the high value placed on professional knowledge, the use of an outside consultant must be carefully approached. Key nursing groups will need to be involved in consultant selection, perhaps through informal interviews, in order that uncertainty about expertise is dispelled at the beginning. Otherwise, a tendency to distrust outsiders will limit the nursing organization's ability to apply the information provided by such experts.[12]

The more sophisticated the actual technology associated with a new structure, the greater the need for support personnel. The presence of technology introduces complex and numerous line-staff relationships. Therefore, the time needed for successful change is increased as well as the complexity of the change project itself.

Authority

Professional organizations have been described as possessing a dual authority structure: management and professional.[13] When nursing organizations are considering the implementation of change, this unique feature must be examined during project selection. Otherwise, authority conflicts will arise and impede implementation when authority is blurred.

The negative effects of authority issues can be minimized by selecting a project in which decision-making points are clearly identified and assigned to management, staff, or both. When information about project status is presented, it is identified as information only or information requiring action. When professional knowledge is required for management decisions regarding project implementation, processes for participation and delegation must be in place.[14]

Dual authority structures are particularly problematic for middle managers in nursing. These individuals are the most likely persons to be caught in a conflict between professional and organizational needs.[15] The use of middle manager liaisons or networking groups during the restructuring project cycle will minimize some of this conflict through dialogue and sharing of solutions.

Hierarchy and its related status requirements accompanies dual authority structures. This feature of professional organizations creates difficulties in the implementation of new nursing structures because of fears of lost status. Perceived threats to power or influence will result in significant organizational resistance to the change if left unaddressed. The project selected will need to assure that the existing reward structure matches the performance demands of the new structure. In addition, top nursing management must be required to change along with the rest of the nursing organization. This means systems need to be designed that detect when top managers are not supporting the change. At the same time, nursing leaders must take care to not over-focus on these individuals to the neglect of the group or the organization.[16]

Complexity

Professional organizations are usually complex, encompassing multiple nursing specialties and many interdisciplinary relationships. This specialty focus results in a tendency for work groups to become isolated from each other. Consequently., although specialty programs can be successfully implemented by individuals, organization-wide change requires a degree of cooperation that is probably not present in the beginning stages of the restructuring cycle. Effective project selection and design recognizes the cooperation/collaboration requirements of proposed structures.

As nursing organizations increase in size and complexity, behavior tends to replicate itself and become more centralized within a division. Interdependencies among other professional groups are jealously guarded. The isolation of nursing work groups from one another may result in considerable conflict. For example, labor and delivery nurses may rarely interface with critical care nurses. When they do (usually when a maternity patient is admitted to critical care), professional disagreements occur because of varying procedures, differences in the degree of standardization, and because of differences in primary focus. In addition, divisions of labor and accompanying differences in specialty focus may create significant interdepartment competition for scarce resources, recognition, or acceptance of a particular world view.[17]

Differences in the rationale and need for change, competition for scarce resources, varying world views, and differing autonomy needs represent complexity-related barriers to the collaboration needed for successful project implementation. However, there are ways to design a restructuring project so that diversity becomes a strength rather than a weakness. This is discussed in further detail in the planning section of this book.

Environment

Much has been written in the literature about the organizational culture and its influence upon nurses. Two features of the organizational environment are particularly relevant for nursing organizations considering the introduction of a major change: power and hostility.

Inaccurate or incomplete identification of power relationships during the implementation of new structures will result in certain failure. There are some tough questions to answer. Who has the power to block or to influence the restructuring initiative? Who holds the financial purse strings? Will there be the necessary support to deal with the roadblocks of backlash-resistant cynicism and the fatigue accompanying most change? What will the proposed new structures do to existing power relationships?

The introduction of any change reinforces our awareness of the limitations in individual power.[18] This awareness may be even more intensified in highly competitive organizations, where the winners of corporate favor battle their weaker foes. As change unfolds, strategies must be carefully chosen so that premature information and/or expectations do not create alarm and feelings of powerlessness.

The larger and more complex an organization, the sharper the distinctions between managers and staff. Management roles become critical linkages for such nursing organizations.[19] Strong distinctions between staff and managers creates a two-tiered information system as well as a leveled authority structure. Individual managers will differ in the amount and the quality of the information shared with staff. This can result in the lack of timely and accurate information, rumors, uncertainty, and resistance to the new structures. The project eventually selected will include limitations upon the time lags between the sharing of project information, new role education, and their required behavioral expression.[20] In this way, it will be clear to managers when, how, and what information needs to be shared at key stages during implementation.

Clearly, the diversity of complex organizations requires that restructuring projects be designed in order that everyone affected has the opportunity to agree with the change. This approach is time-consuming, requires significant interface and dialogue, and can be very frustrating, but is well worth the time devoted to such activities.

Power imbalances are simply a natural feature of any nursing organization. One clinical service may have more experts on the proposed change or more people interested in participating than another service. These groups may dominate the decision making. Approaches to this dilemma are critical. Nursing groups participating in the change need to be evaluated for the presence of resources and personal commitment. Those lacking such advantages will require more work, and perhaps the sharing of resources from services that already have them. In addition, those in a position to publicly communicate about the status of the change must studiously avoid comparisons.

The importance of administrative influence and support cannot be ignored in any discussion of power. The project selected must be able to gain the commitment of those individuals who genuinely identify with the new structure and who are willing to stake their futures on its success. During implementation, opportunities for feedback regarding the environmental responses to the change are essential to the detection of potential erosion of support. Nursing leaders must make sure that they surround themselves with individuals representing a diversity of viewpoints, so that a diversity of feedback is ensured.

Administrative support for a restructuring project will remain strong to the extent that coalitions are successfully managed. Support for the new nursing structure must be carefully marketed to the rest of the organization. An interactive monitoring of the environment, including repetitious presentations of the same information to various professional groups and evaluation of their concerns, needs to be built into the project design.

Hostility

Finally, hostility is a dimension of professional organizations that must be examined for its influence upon project selection. Organizations range from pleasant to hostile environments. Hostility is usually strong when an organization is facing a crisis. Extreme hostility in any environment drives an organization to centralize its structure, even temporarily. This is because tight supervision reduces time spent on arguing or trying to reach consensus. Unfortunately, many decisions to restructure come out of a crisis situation. When organizations face a crisis such as a unionization attempt or a financial shortfall, a hostile environment emerges in which distrust is high, people criticize each other for mistakes, and groups keep to themselves unless it is absolutely necessary to come together. The typical organizational response is to centralize decision making so that time is reduced in arguing, authority for decisions is clear, and one person makes most of the decisions. However, this approach is in direct contradiction to the need for decentralization so that the new structure is well understood and supported. Eventually, the tension between the need to decentralize/centralize communications and decision making contributes not only to project failure but also to the demise of the organization itself.[21] Clearly, the introduction of new structures in highly unstable or crisis environments is not recommended.

MOTIVATIONS OF INDIVIDUALS AND GROUPS

Individuals and groups change themselves through conscious actions and decisions. Proposed solutions are examined in relationship to the unique motivations of each individual and nursing group, as well as the proximity of critical groups to the change itself. The project eventually selected will be designed in order to maximize motivational factors.

In addition, other professional groups, including physicians, administrators, other department heads, social workers, and pharmacists must be identified according to their proximity to the change. Then planning and implementation strategies can be applied in order to assure cooperation and support. For example, department heads may wonder who they will talk to about nursing practice concerns, if a product line management structure eliminates the head nurse role. If these concerns are not planned for and addressed, significant resistance and perhaps loss of needed resources could be the result.

Nursing groups at the center of a restructuring project are struggling to acquire the new sets of behaviors required for successful changes, while those less involved talk about the new structure and wonder how it will eventually influence their own work lives. Both groups need to be addressed in the planning and evaluation stages of the project cycle. Mismatching group characteristics and intervention strategies can make for a perilous course.

For the groups most influenced by the implementation of a new nursing structure, re-education, tolerance for resistance, and experimentation with new behaviors are appropriate change strategies in the early phases. Comfort with the new order begins to emerge as individuals and groups have successful experiences. By midimplementation, groups can be encouraged to suspend judgment and experiment, without risking that the experiments will become permanent. After extensive experimentation and evaluation, the new structure will be adopted. The adoption of a new nursing structure by the most involved nursing groups signals that the change is ready to be formalized in job descriptions, performance standards, and policy and procedure. Once these elements are developed and approved, the new nursing structure is said to be accepted by the whole organization.[22]

Those groups not directly involved need frequent communication about the progress of the change and about implications for their own futures. In addition, opportunity for contact between involved and noninvolved groups enhances understanding about the change and keeps rumors from getting out of hand.

Not only do groups vary in their response to change, but individual professional nurses also demonstrate unique differences in their readiness to adopt a new nursing structure and its requisite behavior requirements. Rogers (1983) describes the process of change as a transformation whereby networks of individuals in organizations engage in a person-to-person exchange in the adoption of an innovation. Proposed solutions and their implementation should be examined so the project that maximizes individual motivations is the one that is selected and designed.

The first nursing group to become excited about a new nursing structure are the risk-takers in the organization. They thrive on new ideas and are comfortable with uncertainty. Because they are always seeking opportunities to improve the status quo or to learn something new, these nurses can be easily perceived as major irritants to the organization. Clinical nurse specialists sometimes are the predominant members of the risk-taking group, although staff nurses, managers, and other professionals can certainly be found there as well. The function of the risk-taking group in the adoption of a new nursing structure is to build awareness and amplify understanding.[23] The project selected should enhance the role of risk-takers. For example, this group might do the initial reading about the change and provide the initial education programs about the proposed new structure. Such involvement will carry their excitement and their enthusiasm across the organization.

Unfortunately, the risk-takers cannot carry a change alone in a nursing organization. Often, they are viewed as outside the norm. In order for ideas to move into action the "respected opinion leaders"[24] must emerge as supporters of the restructuring project. These nurses can successfully champion the adoption of a new idea because they are respected for their clinical knowledge and skills, their advocacy on behalf of other nurses, and their influence across the organization. These nurses are indeed the pioneers in the adoption of a new structure. They will experience pressure from their more conservative colleagues and will need the continued visible support of the nursing leader. The role of this group is to legitimize the new nursing structure as an important and necessary change for the nursing organization.

The influence of opinion leaders results in an early majority who are committed to the new structure. Momentum builds when this nursing group commitment occurs, along with pockets of support.[25] However, the new structure will not yet be seen as a legitimate form for nursing work. Nurses in the early majority will be talking to one another. To the extent that their experiences are positive, increased experimentation, abandonment of history, and excitement about the change will spread throughout the organization. The reverse relationship is also true. Errors in design and implementation must be watched for closely. Nurses must be encouraged to share bad experiences with the new structure, so that critical evaluation and necessary modifications can follow. Otherwise, the early majority could spread news of the project failure.

The last two groups to become committed to the new structure are the "late majority" and the "laggards." These groups are the most hesitant about the introduction of anything new. The late majority get involved in response to increased organizational pressure, including peer pressure, for change. The laggards are those individuals who are focused on the past.[26] In nursing organizations, these individuals have usually been employed for a long time and may resent the intrusion of newcomers with new ideas. They are limited in their vision and will fight the change at every turn. Prior to planning, those individuals within the nursing organization who have the most difficulty with change, along with those groups with whom they have the most influence, must be identified. Unfortunately, top nursing management groups are the places where "laggards" may be found. The project selected and its accompanying interventions should be designed so that these individuals are not put into leadership positions.

If potential resistors are not identified, the progress and outcomes of implementation are jeopardized. For example, one nursing organization implementing shared governance struggled with the development of a nursing practice council for over one year. The council was made up of a mix of nurses from all levels and all departments of the nursing organization. The council could never seem to make a decision, discussion was stilted, and great ambiguity about roles prevailed. There was discussion that shared governance should be abandoned because it was a waste of time. At the end of the year, the nursing manager member was replaced by a younger colleague who had recently joined the organization because of its move to shared governance. The new manager member recognized that additional education about the role of the practice council was desperately needed by all. Once this education was completed, the group quickly moved into decision making.

The obstacle was the former nursing manager. She had been assigned to facilitate this group because of her seniority. However, her history of resistance to change, her fears of lost status, and her key position in the nursing hierarchy made it impossible for the group to confront her negative behavior or to ask for what they needed to move forward. If her resistance had been identified in relation to proposed solutions, then planning would have resulted in the implementation of strategies to help her overcome her resistance, if possible.

Each proposed solution must be examined in relation to the management of critical individuals and groups. Planning activities can then assure that the right individuals are involved at the right time in the change process. By carefully placing individuals in key places at certain stages in the restructuring projects, dominant and new coalitions connect to achieve desired results.

LEADERSHIP STYLE

A dilemma confronting the nursing leader during project selection is the need to match the leadership requirements of the new structure to that which already exists in the organization. New nursing structures differ in the degree to which they are revolutionary. The more revolutionary an idea, the more need for what Burn (1978) has described as a transformational leadership style.[27] The transformational leader is able to motivate followers to commit to revolutionary ideas by engaging in intense interpersonal relationships that motivate followers to a higher level of productivity and transform their values to equal those of the leader.[28] Transformational leaders have a clear vision of the future, and can make compelling arguments for the support of the followers. Such leaders are able to maintain the vision when the going gets rough. Also, the followers of such a leader feel empowered to work to their potential and encouraged to be responsible and accountable. Finally, transformational leaders are often organizational teachers. They see mistakes as opportunity for learning, which in turn encourages experimentation and risk-taking.[29] The relationship between leaders and followers is mutually respectful and interdependent.

The magnet hospital studies give support to the strong role that a transformational leadership style can play. In most of the organizations, the top nursing leaders employed such a style and were often recognized nationally for their professional vision.[30] The more transformational the leadership style of the top nursing leader, the more easily a revolutionary idea is introduced and supported.

However, there is evidence that there needs to be a blend of the transformational and transactional leadership styles within an organization, for both seem to have their place. As opposed to a transformational leadership style, some nursing leaders use transactional styles. The transactional leadership style is based upon exchanges rather than interpersonal connectedness. Followers are given something in return for what the leaders need, usually to fulfill the mission of the organization. Effective transactional leaders are able to accurately assess followers' needs and then find a way to meet the demands. These leaders know what actions must be taken in order for subordinates to achieve the right outcome.[31]

In the implementation of new nursing structures, there is a need for both styles but at different times in the process. The transformational leadership style should be used in the introduction of the new structure in order to gain commitment and at those key points in implementation when commitment needs renewal. On the other hand, the transactional leadership style is important when new nursing roles are introduced in the organization. Through their skills in the assessment of individual needs and their working knowledge of subordinate strengths and weaknesses, transactional leaders clarify role confusion and identify the functions necessary for successful performance within the new structure.

In determining which project will be selected for implementation, the leadership demands of each proposal should be carefully evaluated and then matched with the styles of nurses in leadership positions across the organization. A revolutionary idea needs more transformational leadership than one that is simply an advancement of a structure that is already in place.

Clinical nursing and nursing management leaders may differ in style because of the developmental nature of leadership skills. Some leaders, due to a lack of mentoring or experience, may operate out of a low transactional level based predominantly upon meeting personal agendas. They assume that all people operate that way. They may aspire to a higher level of transaction but are unable to participate with subordinates and engage in the mutuality needed for higher level transactions.[32] This type of leadership style is most dangerous at the top and middle management level, because such individuals are not able to motivate followers to commitment beyond self-interests.

At the next level of transactional leadership, individuals can consider both their own needs and the needs of subordinates. They are able to treat subordinates as individuals. Some subordinates need the concrete payoff of personal need satisfaction while others are motivated by recognition and mutual valuing by the leader. This transactional leader is the most effective because the focus is on the communication of positive values, including commitment, fairness, loyalty, and respect. The leader-subordinate relationship differs from that of the transformational leader in that the goals and values of the subordinate remain unchanged.[33] However, this style has many features of transformational leadership and may be a transitional stage skill.

Nursing leaders interested in examining the leadership leading to the acquisition of transformational leadership styles of key nursing leaders prior to the introduction of a new nursing structure can use the Multifactor Leadership Questionnaire developed by Bass (1984).[34] The possible types of transactional leadership and their relationship to transformational leadership are illustrated in Figure 2-2.

THE ULTIMATE RESOURCE: NURSING MANAGEMENT EXPERTISE

The introduction of new nursing structures requires significant nursing management knowledge and skill at all levels of the nursing organization. Unfortunately, many nursing organizations suffer from a lack of expertise because the best nursing clinicians are the individuals who are promoted into key management positions. Such individuals may find it very difficult to ask for help or to even return to school because they feel that they will lose face. After all, as senior managers they should know what course to pursue.

Potential new structures should be examined for their demands upon management expertise. For example, the implementation of shared governance structures requires comfort with letting go of clinical skills accompanied by increased involvement in management roles and

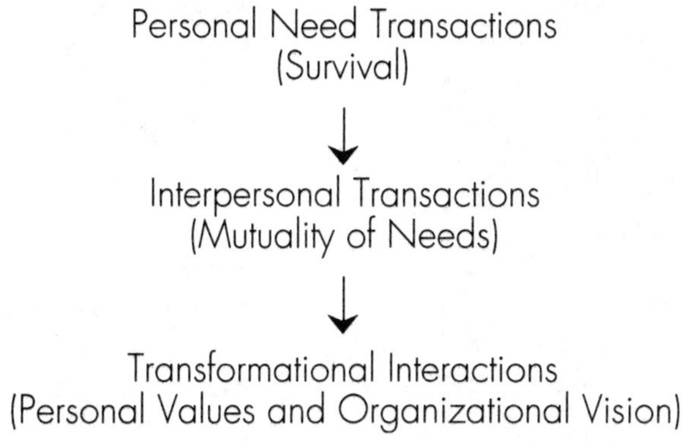

Figure 2-2 Types of Transactional/Transformational Leadership Styles. *Source:* Information from *Academy of Management Review*, Vol. 12, No. 4, pp. 648–657, Academy of Management, © 1987.

functions. Managers not possessing the necessary expertise to move into expanded management roles will resist the transition. In addition, incorrect decisions may be made about which problems require management decisions versus those requiring clinical or staff decisions. Outdated operational systems, left unaddressed because of a lack of expertise, will negatively color the performance of new delivery systems.

Exhibit 2-1 Elements of an Organizational Assessment

Organizational Structure

- authority roles
- degree of formalized rules and procedures
- centralized/decentralized decision making
- divisions of labor
- number and type of interdisciplinary relationships
- age
- complexity
- sophistication of technology

Organizational Processes

- communication style and processes
- decision-making style
  —participative
  —group participating
- quality of information
- coordination practices
  —RN/RN
  —RN/other professionals
  —manager/RN
  —manager/other professionals
- leadership styles
- integrating mechanisms

Group Relationships

- autonomy
- conflict/cooperation
- competition
- commitment to excellence
- openness to innovation
- motivations of target individuals and groups
- degree of differences in specialization

Authority

- financial
- formal position
- professional
- transformational/transactional
- bureaucratic

Environment

- hostile/pleasant
- power relationships
- administrative support
- management philosophy

Resources

- time
- money
- technical knowledge and expertise
- level of nursing management expertise
- sophistication of nursing administrative systems

Considerable planning skills are essential early in the project selection, while directing, controlling, and evaluating are needed later. In addition, the implementation of a new structure is impeded if the necessary administrative systems are not in place. Information systems, reporting systems, acuity systems, integration with the entire health care organization, educational resources, and effective problem solving vary according to management expertise. Nursing leaders interested in evaluating their administrative structure and processes for expertise are advised to apply the Standards of Organized Nursing Services, published by the American Nurses Association.

CONDUCTING AN ORGANIZATIONAL ASSESSMENT

Specifying the organizational requirements for the introduction of a new nursing structure is the central theme of the project selection stage. The elements of a comprehensive organizational assessment are listed in Exhibit 2-1. If there is a match between the desired structure and organizational requirements, the restructuring cycle moves into a formal planning stage. If there is not a match, a decision to not change at this point of time is appropriate. Instead, work to minimize organizational obstacles in preparation for a future implementation would be in order.

NOTES

1. Frame, J.D. (1987). *Managing Projects in Organizations*. San Francisco: Jossey-Bass Inc., Publishers, p. 8.
2. Ibid., pp. 16–19.
3. Adizes, I. (1988). *Corporate Life Cycles*. Englewood Cliffs, NJ: Prentice-Hall, Inc., pp. 161–163.
4. Ibid., p. 167.
5. Ibid., p. 168.
6. Zaltman, S. and Duncan, R. (1977). *Strategies For Planned Change*. New York: John Wiley & Sons, p. 263.
7. Ibid., p. 279.
8. Benveniste, G. (1987). *Professionalizing The Organization*. San Francisco: Jossey-Bass Inc., Publishers, p. 39.
9. Mintzberg, H. (1979). *The Structuring of Organizations*. Englewood Cliffs, NJ: Prentice-Hall, Inc., p. 374.
10. Ibid., pp. 373–374.

11. Mintzberg, H. (1979). pp. 363–365.
12. Ibid., p. 375.
13. Benveniste (1987), pp. 59–72.
14. Ibid., pp. 74–85.
15. Stevens, B. (1985). *The Nurse As Executive.* Gaithersburg, MD: Aspen Publishers, Inc., pp. 244–247.
16. Zaltman, G. and Duncan, R. (1977), p. 21.
17. Ibid., pp. 76–77.
18. Moss Kanter, R. (1989). *When Giants Learn To Dance.* New York: Simon & Schuster, pp. 64–67.
19. Stevens, B. (1985), pp. 244–245.
20. Zaltman, G. and Duncan R. (1977), p. 30.
21. Mintzberg, H. (1977), pp. 281–282.
22. Rogers, E. (1983). *Diffusion Of Innovations.* New York: The Free Press, pp. 10–34.
23. Ibid., p. 248.
24. Ibid., p. 248.
25. Ibid., p. 249.
26. Ibid., pp. 249–250.
27. Burns, J.M. (1978). *Leadership.* New York: Harper & Row Publishers.
28. Singer, M.S. and Singer A.E. (1986). Relation between transformational vs. transactional leadership preference and subordinates personality: An exploratory study. *Perceptual and Motor Skills,* 62(2), 775–780.
29. Bennis, W. and Nanus, B. (1985). *Leaders: The Strategies for Taking Charge.* New York: Harper & Row Publishers.
30. Kramer, M. and Schmolenberg, C. (1988). Magnet hospitals: Part I: Institutions of excellence. *Journal of Nursing Administration,* 18(4), 13–24.
31. Singer, M. (1985). Transformational vs. transactional leadership: A study of New Zealand company managers. *Psychological Reports,* 57(3), 143–146.
32. Kuhnart, K.W. and Lewis P. (1987). Transactional and transformational leadership: A constructive/developmental analysis. *Academy of Management Review,* 12(4), 648–657.
33. Ibid., p. 653.
34. Bass, B. (1984). *Leadership and Performance Beyond Expectations.* New York: The Free Press.

CHAPTER 3

Planning for the Implementation of New Nursing Structures

Formal planning follows the selection of a nursing structure that is believed to remedy identified problems. Much has been written about the need for planning, but few organizations do it very well. Effective planning provides clarity in the midst of uncertainty and creates opportunities for controlling and monitoring the actual implementation.

The project plan is a road map that tells everyone how the organization will get from step A to step B. It is the culmination of all the work that has gone before, including the identification of needs, the selection of a new structure, and the clarification of resources to be allocated to implementation and maintenance.

The planning stage is where the specification of the new structure occurs, along with the delineation of activities needed for implementation. Effective planning infuses the organization with a proactive stance towards change. Implementation needs are anticipated and methods for assuring that what was planned is actually happening are outlined in great detail.[1] A well-defined plan for restructuring is the result of the nursing organization thinking the problem through. It should change as circumstances change.

Planning provides the necessary discipline for nursing organizations to reduce a tendency to react rather than plan. This tendency is replaced with the purposeful reordering of structures and processes through the planning process.[2]

DEFINITIONS OF PLANNING

Planning is a process that allows a nursing organization to come to an agreement about a given set of details about the future. Time dimensions are put around the selected restructuring project, allowing for the acquisition of new role expectations and the learning that accompanies them.[3]

Effective planning operationalizes the project concept and definitions in a very specific manner, reducing uncertainty and ambiguity about the future. Matching is achieved by adequately assessing the organization in relation to resources. Matching will be successful if the data base upon which decisions are made is adequate.[4]

The focus of the planning phase is to identify those factors that are amenable to change. However, there are unexpected internal and external events that will have an impact upon goal achievement. To the extent that these occurrences can be predicted and integrated into planning, potential negative effects can be moderated.

For example, the external and internal demands to intensify utilization management activities in one organization created significant barriers in the implementation of nursing shared governance. Utilization management activities, by their controlled functions, are experienced as lessening the authority and autonomy of professional groups. Commonly, utilization management activities are not welcomed change. Shared governance structures also alter authority relationships. Clinical nurses experience an increase in authority over their own practice and nursing managers are empowered by their expanded administrative functioning. In this case, nursing leaders knew of the impending changes in utilization management but did not assess how this relationship might affect implementation. Consequently, professional group resistance to nursing shared governance was much stronger than anticipated. It was seen, particularly by physicians, as another encroachment upon already dwindling influence over patient care. Nursing leaders had to delay implementation of the new structure in order to regain administrative support. The influence of new utilization management procedures could have been anticipated in planning and addressed during the organizational preparation for shared governance. Instead, nursing leaders found themselves handling the expressions of resistance from several professional groups. It was not until the planning team sat down and compared notes that the problem was recognized as related to new utilization management procedures. By then, significant barriers to implementation had already developed.

Money, time, and resources (material and human) are some of the "givens" in a restructuring plan. Time schedules assure that implementation is happening as planned and that milestones are reached as identified. Money is handled through the development of a project budget. The ability to control budget variances is directly related to how well the budget is specified during planning. Careful resource allocation assures that the best possible efforts are being made to allocate limited resources to a restructuring project.[5]

Plans are simply the best guesses about the future rather than fact. There is no way to accurately predict what will occur during implementation and how events will eventually unfold to produce the final nursing structure. The infusion of this attitude into the planning process makes necessary or urgent plan modification later on a much more acceptable practice.

In general, the specification of a plan about the future reduces a significant amount of wariness about the change. The degree of detail possible to achieve in any plan is directly related to the amount of uncertainty about the final structure.[6] For example, some new nursing delivery systems have highly predictable and clearly identified implementation steps associated with them, borne of the experience of other users. Some other kinds of restructuring efforts, such as the implementation of a nursing managed care program, are truly pioneering efforts. In such situations, there is no road map. Planning needs to take a staged or phased approach. Implementation occurs in phases, during which time activities are defined and implemented—one phase at a time.[7]

The natural tendency of members of the planning team to bring their own world view to bear constrains the choice of knowledge applied and data selected for analysis. In addition, the tendency of nursing groups to quantify and analyze everything leads to a lack of respect for those things that are not easily understood or quantified. Unfortunately, unexpected turns of events are sure to occur, making total specification and quantification of implementation activities a fruitless endeavor.

Planning must always be considered to be incomplete. This seeming paradox can be reconciled by maintaining two views of planning.

Formal planning processes are applied in order to define those predictable, easily described and supervised events. Informal planning occurs in response to evaluation and the monitoring data collected during implementation.[8]

TYING PLANNING ACTIVITIES TO ORGANIZATIONAL PROBLEM-SOLVING STYLE

Since planning involves considerable problem-solving activities, the restructuring plan that is ultimately developed will reflect the problem-solving styles commonly used by the nursing organization. These may either facilitate or obstruct effective planning. In considering the implementation of new nursing structures, three problems must be addressed: What methods will be used to choose a design for the new structure? How will change activities be defined for implementation? What administrative structure will be developed during implementation? The manner in which these questions are answered is indicative of the problem-solving style(s) used by the nursing organization.

Miles and Snow (1978)[9] outlined four basic problem-solving styles in organizations, as illustrated in Exhibit 3-1.

Before planning begins, the nursing organization's typical problem-solving style must be identified and, if necessary, moderated. A defender style may be comfortable but harm planning by omitting the input of key groups or by missing important activities for implementation. The reactor style is simply dysfunctional, since this style produces inadequate or even inaccurate implementation strategies.

Ginn (1990), in a study of hospital problem solving during the changing environment of the 1980s, found that analyzers were least likely to change their problem-solving approach in response to environmental demands. Over half of the defenders and reactors studied did change to prospectors or analyzers.[10] It may be that the adaptive approach to problem solving has the greatest strength and resilience in the face of change. These approaches to problem solving should be nurtured and developed during the planning process.

THE INFLUENCE OF TRADITION

There exists an institutional memory that is expressed in organizational rituals and traditions.[11] Nurses in organizations tend to put their

Exhibit 3-1 Organizational Problem-Solving Styles. Adapted from Miles and Snow (1978).

Defender
- Enacts upon stable environments with limited alternatives
- Decision making is centralized
- Resource/technology decisions are cost-effective

Prospector
- Constantly searches for new products or services; domain is broad
- New structures are looked upon as short-term to allow flexibility and effective response to changing demands
- Continuous improvement is a philosophy
- A decentralized decision-making structure exists.

Analyzer
- Entrepreneurial organization which searches for improvement while maintaining stability
- Part of the organization is in flux and part is stable
- New structures are both flexible and cost-effective
- Both centralized and decentralized structures for decision making exist

Reactors
- Inconsistent responses accompanied by poorly defined strategies
- Knee jerk responses to environment which fail to consider organizational realities

Source: Information from *Organizational Strategy: Structure and Process* by R.E. Miles and C.C. Snow, McGraw Hill, © 1978.

understanding of a new structure into the context of all that has gone before.

The introduction of a new nursing structure necessarily builds upon the past. Often the same support departments are called upon for assistance. Similarly, when planning groups first come together, they call upon their knowledge of past experiences with change (both good and bad), their expertise in planning for past projects, as well as the stories told about past changes. Listen to the content discussed the next time a planning meeting is convened for its initial session!

Tradition gives meaning, a sense of rightness, and legitimacy. It is an entrenched way of perceiving reality. Because of the strength of tradition, nursing leaders have a very difficult time removing its influence on the present or adapting it to meet current demands.[12]

Mind sets about the world are the individual expression of tradition. They are internalized within individuals and expressed in judgment of their present experience, expectations about the way things are, and in the behaviors expressed in the course of doing one's work. Mind sets organize thinking, feeling, and acting. For most individuals, mind sets also define the criteria for appropriate/inappropriate work behavior.[13]

For example, many nursing organizations restructured to a primary nursing delivery system in the 1970s. In the introduction of a new structure today, nurses will give meaning to the experience of change by recalling those experiences. These memories may or may not be related to their present nursing department. The numerous debates and discussions that warranted the decision to implement primary nursing are long forgotten. What is remembered is the actual decision to change, who was involved, and whether or not the change to primary nursing was a positive experience. These experiences are brought into planning discussions and could, if negative, produce distorted planning decisions.

How can the influence of tradition upon planning decisions be limited? It is necessary, in the very first planning sessions, to become aware of relevant history. This means sorting past change experiences into facts, rumors, and what is unclear or unknown about past changes. Do not accept individual interpretations at face value! Discussion will follow which points out how the present change replicates or differs from past change experiences.

Second, in the daily monitoring of implementation activities, the influence of history is identified and judged helpful or harmful.[14] If harmful, then discussions of history and its relevance to the present change must be repeated.

Finally, the discomfort that arises in the face of change can sometimes be interpreted as the result of challenges to traditional mind sets about the way things should be. Judgment needs to be applied regarding whether or not the discomfort is becoming dysfunctional. If the discomfort is dysfunctional, then sessions to address the conflict between tradition and changes must be scheduled.

PARTICIPATIVE PLANNING

Planning can be conceived of as a political process of consensus building. This participative philosophy allows for the unique needs of subgroups to be heard, and if possible addressed during implementation. Subgroup participation in planning also provides the authority needed to monitor their activities during implementation and extends the rationale of the project throughout the organization.[15] In order to achieve true participation in planning, members from each of the major work groups within the nursing organization should be involved in planning activities.

In particular, first line managers and professional nursing staff need to participate on the planning teams. These individuals can do great harm to implementation if they are not on board. Participation in planning strengthens commitment to successful implementation.

Empowerment in planning partnerships is clear. Nurses will experience an increased access to top nursing management, readily available information about the need for the new nursing structure, and a timely response to questions from fellow planning group members. Participative planning enables individuals to become sources of positive influence for others, because of their understanding of the change and its relationship to the organization's business. The nurses involved in planning have the added responsibility of selling those around them on the advantages of the new structure.[16]

Another benefit of participation is that the professional nursing staff participants are given the opportunity during planning to describe how implementation activities may put pressure on the staff, and how they might interfere with the delivery of quality care.

FORMING MANAGEMENT–STAFF PLANNING PARTNERSHIPS

The development of a truly participative planning process, involving both professional staff and managers, certainly changes internal roles, relationships, and power dynamics. Power is most strongly influenced because a new attitude is required among those managers who feel that participation is a gift bestowed upon the professional staff. Instead, managers and staff are viewed as equal partners, each with something significant to contribute to the planning process. The nursing leader seeking to successfully implement an integrated planning approach must scan the nursing management team for the existence of those maternalistic attitudes that can undermine true partnerships.[17]

PRESSURES OF PARTNERSHIPS

With power comes the accountability to become part of the solution. Newly empowered individuals struggle with the pressures of accountability and responsibility. They had become accustomed to responding to a lack of control in their work life by blaming, complaining, or withdrawing from the organization. These behaviors must now be replaced with objective and meaningful discussions of real solutions with management from all levels in the organization.[18] This can be a difficult shift and requires constant attention by the nursing leader.

There is also a significant change in the role of nursing support staff, such as educators and clinical nurse specialists. Traditionally, these individuals have been given the responsibility for nursing organization program/project development. With the implementation of a participative planning model, their role shifts to one of integrating and coordinating rather than leading or dominating the project.[19] This may be a difficult role for those nurses who sought expanded roles because of a strong drive for independence and a certain impatience with working through others. Participative planning does not allow for such independence.

For all participants in the planning process, integrative skills such as gathering information from multiple sources, overcoming preconceived notions and tradition, active listening to others, and seeking consensus are necessary for success. These skills simply may not have been developed by some. In particular, nurses who are used to presenting their ideas in fully developed packages find it hardest to adjust. Instead, effective planning requires what Moss Kanter (1989) calls the presentation of "half-formed" ideas. Incomplete thinking allows for group input and modification of thoughts. When suggestions are highly structured, suspicion of hidden agendas and fear of manipulation may be generated within the planning group.[20]

The negative reaction of a project group is often a surprise for the structured individual. Most likely, a considerable amount of their time had been spent in developing a detailed plan. The time spent seems to be unappreciated by the group. Also, the reward system is different in a participative planning method. This can be confusing. In the past, structured individuals may have been rewarded for attention to detail and now are receiving negative feedback for the same behavior. It is essential that the nursing leader work with these key individuals so that they do not withdraw their skills from the planning process. Some specification of detail is clearly required during planning, moderated by an emphasis on process and discussion.

A participative planning process is designed to reward participants who are prepared, flexible, frank, and good group participants. In addition, participants need to have a basic value of equity and fair play. Unfortunately, not everyone in a nursing organization embraces this value. Also, in the deliberation of alternatives and actions, competence and incompetence issues are sure to surface. For the professional staff, this means that top management is seen in a more realistic manner and expectations of leaders will shift to match such reality. For some managers and clinical nurse specialists, the demystification of authority may be seen as a significant loss of status.

Finally, self-awareness is an important skill for participants in the planning process. Personalities become more important, because some personalities may obstruct the planning process as participants engage in face-to-face debate.

OPERATIONAL VERSUS PROFESSIONAL GOALS IN PLANNING

For both individuals and groups, several pertinent questions arise during the planning for structure implementation: How will I know it when I see it? How will participation in these activities influence the achievement of my other goals? What will be the outcomes of the new structure of my work? How will I have to change? How will we know it is working? These questions are answered as management and staff jointly define implementation goals and the work needed to attain them.

There are overlapping goals in any planning process. The clinical staff and the profession they represent have goals. The clients served by the professional staff also have goals. Management goals must include the maintenance and protection of those patient care operations that should continue regardless of implementation.

Goals are statements of the specific end points to which all implementation activities are directed. They are future oriented and reflect the concepts identified at the initiation of a change. There are two major categories of goals found within professional organizations: professional and operational.[21]

Professional goals are broad statements, often incorporating the philosophy or mission of the organization. These broad goals motivate staff to participate in the change and mobilize resources. The principal role of professed goal identification in the planning stage is to give legitimacy for implementation.[22] For example, a professed goal in the implementation of professional practice models or shared governance is to give practitioners at the bedside control over their professional practice.

On the other hand, operational goals are the essential interactions necessary for the nursing organization to function efficiently. These specific operational goals serve as road maps for the acquisition of appropriate behavior, particularly the time lag between education for new behavior and when the behavior is expected to be observed.[23] Considering the previous example, an operational goal during the implementation of shared governance might be the maintenance of certain decision-making processes within the nursing department while clinical decision-making processes are placed in the hands of practitioners. This operational goal is vita to the organization's ability to provide quality care during project implementation.

Agreement by management and staff on both the professed and operational goals of the restructuring project is essential to success. Adequately defined professional goals assure that the new structure is implemented within the context of the organizational mission. Nursing profession goals need to be tied to the overall mission of the organization. In this way, organizational resources can be dedicated to implementation and administrative support remains constant.

Achieving consensus on professional goals is not as difficult as agreeing upon operational goals. Operational goals reflect the complex functions and processes accompanying the provision of patient care. Some of these processes cannot be adequately described or specified.[24] However, dropping them from consideration during planning may jeopardize the quality of care.

Excitement over the professional justification of a new structure may result in the overemphasis of professional goals to the detriment of operational goals. This is a significant risk in nursing organizations when nursing management knowledge and skills are inadequate. The overemphasis of the wrong goals can result in considerable organizational dysfunction during implementation. For example, a strong belief in the need of professional nurses to make their own clinical decisions can result in a decision-making structure that excludes practical nurses and nurse aides. In some nursing organizations, this decision can harm the operational goal of coordinating patient care as the result of considerable hostility between staff in the nursing department. In such cases, effective planning will identify implementation strategies that address both professional and operational goals. A decision-making structure can be designed that assigns clinical nursing decisions to nurses and coordination decisions to a group reflecting the mix of the nursing staff.

LINKING THE VISION AND THE REALITY: AN INTEGRATIVE PLANNING MODEL

Planning must be integrative and participative if it is to function effectively. This means that those most affected by the change are involved in specifying requirements for implementation. In this way, the ideal goals of the new vision can be integrated with the reality of the work place.

The special needs of professional organizations to reconcile diverse viewpoints has already been discussed. Effective planning, however, requires the reaching of consensus about outcomes and the steps leading to their attainment. How can these opposing needs be reconciled?

Herrick (1990) outlines an integrative planning model that is most helpful to consider when implementing new nursing structure. The model proposes that a maximum number of people be involved in planning, while a limited number make the final planning recommendations. This approach addresses the inefficiency created by large groups while maximizing participation.[25]

Project planning occurs through the work of a project team and planning teams. The project team has one member from each major group affected by the change, plus top administration. The project team has the authority to request work of the planning teams, accept the work completed, or to return it for more study. In addition, the project team implements and monitors the activities they have approved.

The project team has many planning teams assigned to it, which do the actual staff work needed for the design of implementation activities.

There can be as many planning teams as needed. In this way, the various interests of diverse groups are reconciled to the common goals of the organization. The teams can do a lot of the groundwork data collection and organizing of information necessary to keep planning focused and to eliminate unnecessary sidetracks. Planning teams engage in implementation proposal development, evaluation plan development, policy definitions, and problem solving.[26]

Both project and planning teams represent a mix of top administration, nursing managers, and professional nursing staff. Necessary support staff should be assigned to groups. These may include nursing educators and specialists, as well as finance staff, personnel staff, information systems staff, and other professional support staff such as social workers and physical therapists. The nature of the project determines which support staff are appropriate for inclusion. Figure 3-1 outlines an example of an integrated planning model in a nursing organization.[27]

The project team is chaired by the vice-president of nursing, who initiated the work on a new delivery system. Other members of the group who approve, implement, and monitor the project include the middle managers who report directly to the top nursing administrator, and representatives from key nursing groups. These key groups may include clinical nurse specialists, head nurses, evening/night supervisors, educators, and staff nurses. Depending upon the significance of the changes being implemented, key department heads such as personnel or finance may be members of the project team.

The middle managers also act as the representatives of the vice-president of nursing on the small planning teams. In this way, top nursing administration's viewpoints are represented in planning team discussions and the potential for proposal veto by the project team is reduced.[28] A chairperson may or may not be appointed to facilitate the work of the planning teams. This is necessary, in particular, if there are numerous small planning teams. If appointed, the chair of planning teams also functions as a member of the project team.

In the redesign of a delivery system, planning teams are comprised of experts in the designated areas along with top management representatives and representatives of the professional staff and key support staff. Professional nurses from different service areas and varying shifts can serve as planning committee members. In addition to stimulating commitment to the project, this diverse participation enables planning members to develop a more global and a longer term view of the deliv-

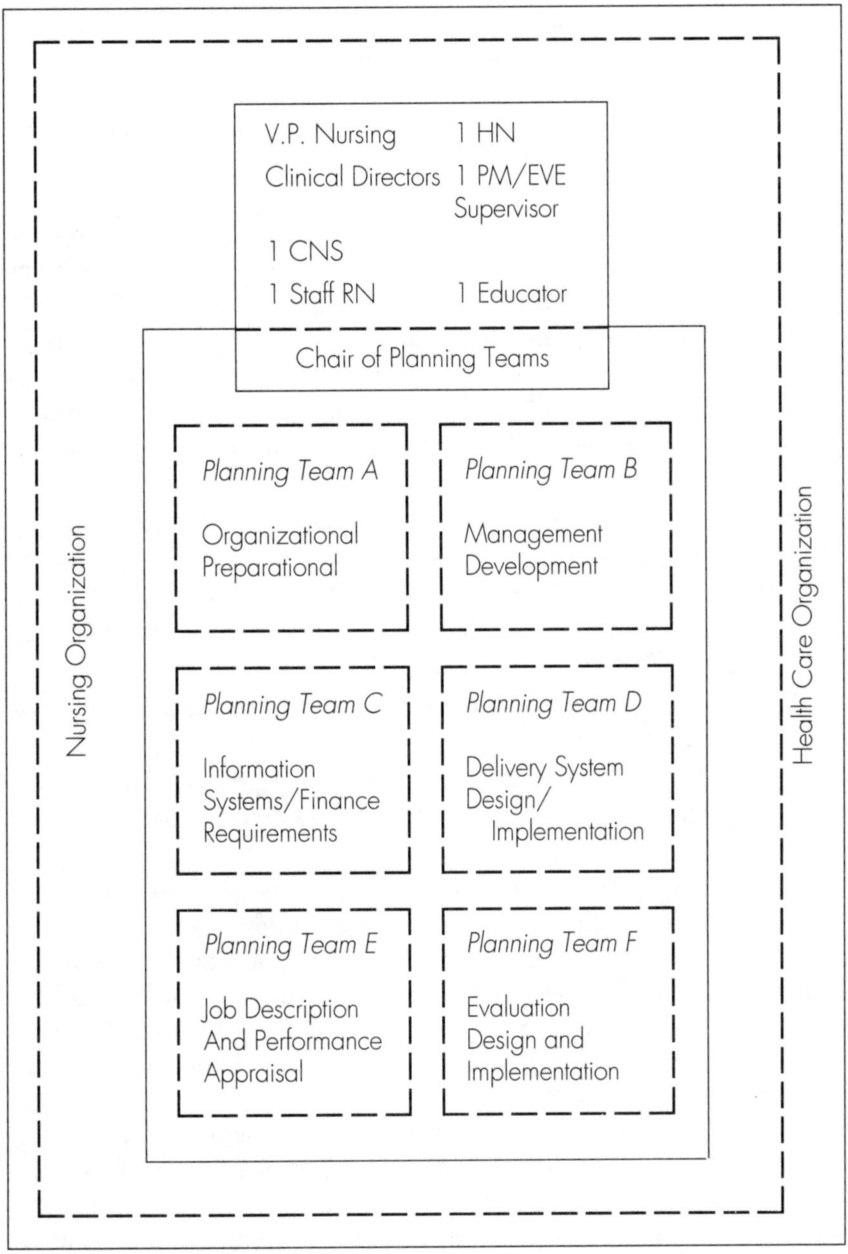

Figure 3-1 Sample Integrated Planning Model for a Delivery System Redesign. *Source:* Adapted from *Joint Management and Employee Participation* by N. Herrick, p. 222, with permission of Jossey-Bass Publishers, © 1990.

ery system change. Once this perspective is achieved, planning teams quickly move into preventative problem solving by recognizing problems early and recommending solutions.[29]

In the delivery system example of Figure 3-1, planning teams are given the following responsibilities:

1. *Organizational Preparation*—Planning and scheduling the communications required to assist key groups in understanding the change and the timetable for implementation.
2. *Management Development*—Identifying management skills required for implementation and providing management education if necessary. Delineating expectations of managers during implementation, including time frames for manager behavioral changes.
3. *Operations*—Planning for operational needs during implementation, including information systems, accounting department function changes and communication requirements.
4. *New Structure*—Designing the new delivery system, specifying implementation steps and schedule.
5. *Personnel*—Developing new job description and performance appraisals along with date of implementation.
6. *Evaluation*—Creating the evaluation design and methodology. Scheduling for baseline, midpoint, and final evaluation points.

The role of the top nursing administrator is crucial to the success of an integrative planning model. The nursing administrator must meet alone, on a regular basis, with the leader of the planning teams as well as the leader of the project team. Along with the establishment of trust and mutual support, these meetings can provide the nursing administrator with important information about the adequacy of resources and the performance of support staff.[30]

Who should lead the project and the planning teams? In many cases, the top nursing administrator prefers to lead the project team, although in some organizations an associate administrator is given this accountability. The nursing leaders responsible for managing the teams must have strong group facilitation skills in order to nurture the development of inherently tentative management-professional staff-support staff partnerships. These skills will assure that the decisions of the project and the planning groups are moved through the organization during implementation.[31]

This is deceptively difficult work and requires that team leaders, particularly those in clinical positions, are freed from some of their regular duties in order to assume the leadership responsibilities. Some of the obstacles to true planning partnerships are described in Exhibit 3-2.

Project and action teams must be carefully planned. Several issues should be considered. First, how will members be assigned to action and project groups? Representatives of all of the work groups in the nursing organization need to be included in planning. Members of the nursing administration team should be assigned to teams. Head nurses

---

Exhibit 3-2 Barriers to Planning Partnerships. Adapted from Moss Kanter (1989).

1. Strategic shifts which occur and the plan must be abandoned or another initiative must take precedent. The reasons for the partnership must be renegotiated. Participants may be replaced or added in order to meet new demands.
2. Differing levels of commitment due to basic differences in skill level, knowledge, and experience.
3. Power imbalances because of varying levels of technical and relationship skills.
4. Power differences when some partners are perceived to have more benefits from the change as compared to others.
5. Conflicting loyalties between what the group wants and what is best for the organization.
6. Poor organization and facilitation of partnership relationships.
7. Inadequate resources assigned to planning. What was initially promised is not delivered, or support staff perform poorly.
8. Conflicts over authority and scope of decision making cause conflict within the planning team.
9. The new structure is not explained well nor adequately tied to the business of the nursing organization.
10. Internal politics among members of the nursing organization are brought into planning, including fears of loss of power, turf battles and competition for administrative recognition.

Source: Information from *When Giants Learn to Dance* by R. Moss Kanter, Simon and Schuster, © 1989.

are more numerous, so slots should be assigned for the head nurses recommended by their colleagues. The same approach is used for the professional nursing staff. Support staff are assigned based on the requirements of the work.[32] Finance, human resource, risk management or quality assurance staff, along with clinical nurse specialists, educators, and other professional groups such as social workers may be essential resources for effective planning.

It is imperative that along with assignment to a team, clear role definitions and delineation of expected behavior are available to all staff so that the appropriate action is taken. In addition, administrative support in the form of meeting arrangement, minute preparation, and preparing calls to meeting must be available to team leaders.

The assignment of support personnel keeps power balances equal between managers (who have access to such staff) and the professional staff (who do not have access to such support). In this way, both groups are able to participate as equal partners. Also, progress is not slowed by the group needing to address administrative details.[33]

PLANNING AS DIRECTION AND CONTROL

A well-defined plan provides management with additional information links to the professional nursing staff. If the plan is designed properly, managers can use it as a tool for directing behavior change and for monitoring implementation.

An advantage of planning over direct supervision is that today's reality is replaced into a timed and future context. Certain current practices become less relevant and the focus shifts to what to do instead. This shift reduces the effectiveness of self-justification and blame as expressions of resistance.[34]

The plan must specify when new behaviors are to be introduced, experimented with, and then formalized into job descriptions and performance expectations. As the plan is communicated throughout the organization, performance expectations are made clear. In addition, time is set aside for learning from errors, promoting a trusting environment.

The purpose of controlling activities is to keep implementation on track. What is actually happening in the organization is compared to what was planned. It is important to keep a realistic picture of change, and to identify how much variance from the original plan is acceptable.

Clearly, in restructuring projects where there are no road maps, more variance is expected. The complexity, size, degree of unpredictability of a project, and unique characteristics of an organization determine the degree of control necessary.[35]

The assignment of project dimensions then leads to the selection of scheduling tools, to guide the direction and control of the project. Responsibility charting, Gantt charting, and PERT (Program Evaluation and Review Technique) are scheduling devices that enjoy much attention in nursing and business literature. These methods are quite popular, and each brings particular strengths and weaknesses to the planning process. The selection of a scheduling tool should be guided by the following questions:

1. Does the tool delineate both tasks and time frames for achievement?
2. Is it clear when activities begin and end?
3. Can varying authority for different types of decisions be integrated with task and time?
4. Will the delay in one set of activities be reflected in the time of other sets? Are activities integrated?
5. Is there a software program which includes the scheduling features necessary for this project?

ORGANIZING PLANNING ACTIVITIES

There are essentially four major classifications of activities that need to be included in a plan and scheduled:

- activities that control obstacles and barriers and maximize organizational strengths
- change strategies aimed at individuals and groups
- the delineation of the actual steps required of a new structure and
- stages of evaluation and its accompanying methodologies.

Change strategies can be further divided into clusters or "tracks"[36] of activities and then scheduled with appropriate responsibility and authority for implementation. The tracks essential for the implementation of shared governance are illustrated in Exhibit 3-3.

Exhibit 3-3 Some Sample Implementation Tracks for the Introduction of Shared Governance

Culture Activities
- Introduction of concept to managers
- Introduction of concept to key clinical nursing leaders
- Integration of change with an existing, functional participative activity
- Preparation of hospital administration
- Preparation of human resources

Management Education Activities
- Assessment of management skills in the top administrative team
- Corrective education to address skill deficiency
- Self-assessment and personal education plans requested of all managers
- Identification of new management skills required by the new structure
- Delineation of behaviors expected of managers in order to facilitate change

Structure Strategies
- Delineation of roles, functions, and memberships of governance councils
- Development of nursing by-laws
- Time lines for council implementation

Reward Systems
- Rewards identified for new competencies
- Integration of shared governance work into performance appraisals and promotion procedures
- Establishment of new forms of recognition

Evaluation Activities
- Acquisition of research expertise and technology
- Development of evaluation design
- Establishment of time lines

The culture track, the management skills track, and the team building track are implemented first. These activities comprise the work of preparing the organization for the introduction of a new structure. The strategy-structure track and the reward system track then follow. These two tracks are concerned with activities that alter the organization's systems and processes. The introduction of new technology, policy and procedure modification, shifting resources, the introduction of new authority structures, and performance program changes are included in this set of activities. Activities for each track are carefully delineated and then scheduled for a certain time frame.[37]

Pilot Units

A decision about pilot units must be made prior to initiation of activities. The initial decision is whether or not to use pilot units to maximize the strength of professional differences, by encouraging experimentation. Organization-wide change may be selected in order to gain standardization and avoid fragmentation of efforts. If pilot units are to be used, certain criteria must be applied in their selection.

Successful pilot units have a history of stable leadership, a successful track record with previous changes, the availability of technical expertise, and credibility within the nursing organization. Sometimes pilot units are chosen because they have the strongest needs for improved structures. Some are selected because they are isolated and failure will not be felt by the rest of the organization. When these reasons determine the choice of a pilot unit, the risk is high that the rest of the organization will not find the change relevant or credible.[38]

If pilot units are identified, planning must address the spread of the new structure to other parts of the organization.[39] Individuals from the pilot unit become important communicators of not only the outcome of change but the experience of it as well.

PITFALLS IN PLANNING

Several obstacles to effective planning can be modified with careful assessment and appropriate intervention. Some plans are not translated in user-friendly terms. Abstract concepts, technical language, or poorly articulated definitions lead to confusion and consequently limit commitment.

Some plans are never used as a change strategy by themselves. Neatly detailed plans sit on the shelves of those who prepared them. Missed opportunities for education and direction are the outcomes of this habit. Plans should be presented, in formal and informal sessions, to all of the key groups. These sessions should be repeated as often as needed, particularly when plan modification is necessary.

Personnel issues can create havoc for effective planning. Clearly, a change in top nursing leadership may alter commitment to the plan entirely. Also, support staff conflicts may arise and block progress on goal attainment. These conflicts are more apt to occur when integrative planning is used as a method and must be appropriately managed.

Planning teams may be assigned activities that are traditionally the scope of a support department. For example, a planning group may be assigned the work of writing new job descriptions for a delivery system. Personnel department staff, who are uncomfortable with this work being done outside the department, may try to sabotage the work of the planning team. Necessary information is delayed. Job descriptions take a long time to be graded. Personnel staff work behind the scenes to divert resources away from the planning team and raise petty objections to performance system modifications.[40]

The interventions required to stop sabotage are very clear. If the top nursing administrator is meeting regularly with planning team leaders, then the development of these turf battles can be identified early. Hospital administrative support for the assignment of support department resources to project planning is reconfirmed. Role expectations of support staff are reiterated with department heads and their staff.

Another pitfall in planning is the nature of the plan itself. As mentioned previously, effective restructuring plans must be both adequate and flexible. Inadequate planning results in project failure or the implementation of a structure that does not meet the identified needs of users. Inflexible plans do not allow for the necessary changes required when circumstances change.

Finally, planning suffers from the existence of hidden agendas. Hidden agendas are a reality of organizational life. However, all efforts must be directed to assure that they have minimum influence upon planning decisions. For example, a nursing administrator may have a hidden agenda to keep the project "under wraps" because of a tentative relationship with the CEO. Similarly, a nursing leader may allow a subordinate to take a visible leadership role in the implementation of a controversial change, in order to avoid risk. Both agendas meet individual needs but create potential harm when administrative support is needed, but not provided, at critical points in the implementation phase.

QUESTIONS TO GUIDE PROJECT PLANNING

1. Which structures/processes are the given targets for change by the new structure?
2. What needs to be included in the project budget?
3. How predictable are the outcomes of the new structure?
4. Can an implementation plan be a long-term plan or must it be a phased plan, 6 months to 1 year at a time?
5. What is the typical problem-solving style engaged in the nursing organization? How will this style influence planning? Does it need to change?
6. How has the nursing organization responded to change in the past? What groups have been involved in past changes? Were past changes successes? How were past changes experienced by individuals and groups? How do past changes influence perceptions of the proposed change?
7. How does the top nursing management team view participation and how is this attitude expressed in behavioral terms? Do attitudes promote true partnerships?
8. Have staff–management partnerships been a common practice for the nursing organization? If not, how will these groups be prepared for partnerships?
9. Can adequate supports be provided for project and planning teams?
10. What is the role of the clinical nurse specialist? the educator? Are role definitions conducive to participation?
11. What professional goals are the basis for new structure implementation? What are the operational goals? How do they relate?
12. How shall the integrated planning process be structured?
13. What internal politics might be brought into planning decisions?
14. What new behaviors are expected of each key nursing group, including top management? How long after education and experimentation with new roles are behaviors expected to be formalized?
15. What scheduling/control tool is best suited for project monitoring and control?
16. How can implementation activities be clustered into tracks?

17. Does the introduction of a new structure require pilot units or organization-wide change?
18. What are the criteria for pilot unit selection?
19. Are the roles of support department staff in planning teams clearly defined and encouraged by department heads?
20. Can any hidden agendas be identified from the way in which planning and implementation activities are delineated?

NOTES

1. Frame, J.D. (1987). *Managing Projects In Organizations.* San Francisco: Jossey-Bass Inc., Publishers, p. 155.
2. Herrick, N. (1990). *Joint Management and Employee Participation.* San Francisco: Jossey-Bass Inc., Publishers, p. 116.
3. Benveniste, G. (1987). *Professionalizing The Organization.* San Francisco: Jossey-Bass Inc., Publishers, p. 117.
4. Fink, S.L., Jenks, R.S., and Willets, R.D. (1983). *Designing and Managing Organizations.* Homewood, Illinois: Richard D. Irwin, Inc., pp. 198–207.
5. Frame, J.D. (1987), p. 156.
6. Ibid., p. 157.
7. Ibid., p. 158.
8. Benveniste, G. (1987), p. 118.
9. Miles, R.E. and Snow, C.C. (1978). *Organizational Strategy, Structure and Process.* New York: McGraw-Hill Book Co.
10. Ginn, G.O. (1990). Strategic change in hospitals: An examination of the response of the acute care hospitals to the turbulent environment of the 1980's. *Health Services Research,* 25(4), 565–591.
11. Kantrow, A.M. (1988). *The Constraints of Corporate Tradition.* New York: Harper & Row Publishers, p. 126.
12. Ibid., p. 163.
13. Ibid., p. 75.
14. Ibid., pp. 87–100.
15. Townsend, M.B. (1990). A participative approach to administrative reorganization. *Journal of Nursing Administration,* 20(2), 11–14.
16. Townsend, M.B. (1990), p. 12.
17. Moss Kanter, R. (1989). *When Giants Learn To Dance.* New York: Simon and Schuster, pp. 141–147.
18. Benveniste, G. (1986), p. 129.
19. Herrick, N. (1990), pp. 124–134.

20. Moss Kanter, R. (1989), p. 154.
21. Benveniste, G. (1986), p. 98.
22. Ibid., pp. 99–100.
23. Ibid., p. 105.
24. Ibid., pp. 100–104.
25. Herrick, N. (1990), p. 25.
26. Ibid., pp. 218–231.
27. Ibid., pp. 221–223.
28. Ibid.
29. Ibid., p. 230.
30. Orth, C.D., Wilkinson, H.E., and Benfau, R.C. (1990). The manager's role as coach and mentor. *Journal of Nursing Administration,* 20(9), 11–15.
31. Ibid., p. 12.
32. Herrick, N. (1990), pp. 231–238.
33. Ibid., p. 238.
34. Benveniste, G. (1987), p. 129.
35. Frame, J.D. (1987), p. 163.
36. Kilman, R.H. (1989). A completely integrated program for creating and maintaining organizational success. *Organizational Dynamics,* Summer, 5–15.
37. Ibid., p. 15.
38. Ibid., p. 13.
39. Ibid., pp. 13–14.
40. Herrick, N. (1990), pp. 237–238.

CHAPTER 4

Managing the Environment during Implementation

This chapter is about the relationship between an organization's environment and the successful introduction of change. Early in the implementation phase, activities must be directed towards stimulating the receptivity of the nursing environment to the new nursing structure. The project team must determine effective implementation strategies for not only tapping the strengths of the nursing environment but also limiting its weaknesses. The culture of the nursing organization and the presence of stressors in the nursing work place are critical elements of the environment demanding intervention before a new structure is implemented. Factors that contribute to cultural problems during implementation include the following:

1. The presence of nursing cultures that either actively or passively reject change.
2. The existence of work place stressors that intensify the stress which normally accompanies change.
3. The development of hysteria or panic from a failure to effectively manage resistance.
4. Status and personality issues that promote maintenance of the status quo.

5. Inadequate or inaccurate education about the new nursing structure.
6. Overlooking the personal and the social relationship aspects of change during implementation.
7. An ineffective communication network that hinders the acceptance of a new structure.
8. Mistakes in the definition of the new nursing roles required by the new nursing structure.
9. Failure to assure the centrality, flexibility, and control over resources of the new nursing structure.
10. Inadequate recognition of the reality of change in a nursing organization.

What are the strategies that can be used by nursing leaders to effectively manage the nursing environment during implementation? A major tool is education. The provision of accurate and complete information about the change to all people affected by the new nursing structure will influence the amount of opposition to the change, both from internal and external sources. Also, education affects the ability of nurses to utilize the new structure appropriately. Accurate information about the change helps nurses to determine what performance is required under the new structure.

Another set of activities involves the implementation of the structure itself. The careful delineation of the actual steps of structure development serves to enhance acceptance and understanding. In addition, the phased introduction of a new structure assures that its features will successfully integrate into the rest of the organization.

Finally, success will be achieved if traditions and rituals are established that signify the importance of the change.

CHARACTERISTICS OF CULTURES

Successful implementation of change is dependent upon whether or not the nursing organization adopts the change as part of its existent culture. The acceptance or rejection of a new nursing structure occurs over time, through a series of actions and choices performed by individuals and groups.[1] The culture influences the acceptance of a new structure. Consequently, the baseline evaluation of the nursing culture is an important step in the early implementation phase.

The assessment of the culture should be designed to examine certain significant issues. What is the nature of the nursing organization's business environment? Are the beds full; is there a staffing shortage or an increase in competition from other providers? Is the health care organization profitable? Is there any anticipation of staff layoffs? What do nursing staff believe about the organization? What are the basic beliefs about health care, nursing, and patient care?

Patient care values and beliefs are expressed in the priority-setting behaviors of nurses, in the documentation of patient care, and in the focus of nursing quality assurance studies. Who are the heroes (past and present) in the nursing organization? Why are they heroes? Are some of their respected behaviors useful to promote in the implementation of new structures or do these behaviors limit success? What traditions exemplify accepted behaviors? What and where are the informal communication systems?[2]

Nursing cultures have some distinct rituals that promote socialization into the culture. Orientation and sophisticated preceptor programs enable the new nurse to identify accepted beliefs and behaviors, and to learn many of the hero stories. However, the increasing numbers of part-time nurses may mean that a substantial portion of the nursing work force is not tuned into the culture. Part-time nurses often have limited orientation and decreased involvement with the culture.[3] Careful attention to the mix of full-time and part-time nurses allows special attention to be focused on the needs of part-time nurses during a major change. If this focus is missing, part-time nurses are at high risk for experiencing significant cultural conflicts. These conflicts stem from not only inaccurate assessment of the culture but from the cultural challenges of the new structure itself!

For example, a newly hired part-time nurse volunteered to be the chair of a new unit quality assurance committee. She was very enthusiastic about the opportunity to participate in quality assurance. Her nursing unit was perceived as a plum assignment because the unit was small and often provided the care for VIP patients. Therefore, many long-term nurses comprised the staff. They had worked very hard to be assigned to this particular unit. There were strong cultural values for maintaining the status quo and avoiding conflict. The part-time nurse found herself rejected by the work group for volunteering, and for taking time away from the unit. After a period of sustained conflict, she eventually left the organization.

This nurse had not been helped to understand the differences between her unit's culture and the culture of the change she was trying to implement. Culture management activities were not included in the implementation plan. If such strategies had been identified, then potential sources of opposition would have been anticipated and limited. In this way, the pioneers of a change project do not become its victims.

Cooke and Lafferty (1989) have described a typology of organizational cultures that has utility when considering the implementation of change.[4] Cultures are classified into three categories: constructive, passive defender, and aggressive defender. The *constructive culture* parallels the culture of excellence. It emphasizes need satisfaction, achievement, creativity, individual growth, participation, and the satisfaction of work groups. The *passive defender culture* forebodes significant resistance to change. It demands the maintenance of the status quo and an avoidance of risk or experimentation. The *passive defender culture* is expressed in behaviors that maintain security needs; assure approval; avoid conflict; emphasize ritual, rules, and tradition; discourage participation, and punish mistakes. Finally, there is the *aggressive defender* culture. This environment produces significant conflicts requiring intervention during implementation, due to power struggles. These conflicts occur because the aggressive defender culture promotes the protection of status and power, rewards confrontation, requires the strict control of subordinates, sets up win–lose relationships, and values perfectionism along with long work hours.[5]

Clearly, the implementation of change demands that the nursing culture be effectively managed. A strong, positive nursing culture prescribes the behaviors necessary for performance in the new structure whereas a weak or negative culture provides obstacles to success. It is difficult to always know which cultural features will support or obstruct a new structure. Valid assessments of the existing culture could be obtained in order to identify and anticipate barriers to successful implementation. Nursing leaders are encouraged to consider the Organizational Culture Inventory (OCI) as a potential tool for such an assessment.[6]

MANAGING STRESS DURING IMPLEMENTATION

Undergoing major reorganization is a major stressor in the nursing environment. The experience of change commonly intensifies the work-related stress already present in the system.[7] Does the nursing staff struggle with staffing shortages and competing demands? Do they complain about a lack of time and/or unclear direction? Do they exhibit symptoms of powerlessness? If these characteristics exist in the work environment, then the introduction of a new structure is experienced as simply another source of stress. Carefully selected implementation activities minimize the potential for overwhelming stress.

A key strategy early in the implementation phase is to assess the nursing organization for existing sources of stress. The next step is to determine the potential of the new structure to put the stress level beyond what can be handled by individuals and groups. Stress is a natural feature of any change but can be intensified to dangerous levels if other significant stressors are already operating in the environment.

Work place generated stress results from demands that exceed the person's ability to handle them.[8] In nursing work, there exists potential for many stressful experiences. Some nursing specialties have an almost overwhelming intensity, such as pediatric oncology or emergency/trauma nursing. In the former, dealing with the death of children on a regular basis is upsetting work. In the latter, too many demands are spilling into the emergency room, at a pace that is almost impossible to keep up with. Nursing groups providing these services may not be appropriate choices for initial pilot units because of the amount of stress generated in the delivery of care.

When implementation does come to high stress areas, it should be accompanied by deliberate methods for reducing the intensity of change. Individual and group social support systems can be provided to staff. The goals of such systems might include stressor identification, legitimizing asking for help as a coping strategy, and the dividing up of implementation work.

A lack of control over one's work is also a stressor for contemporary nurses. Responsibilities may be assigned regardless of an individual's ability. Cumbersome policies, developed with no input from the professional staff, may also make nursing work frustrating and nearly impossible to achieve.

Rules can also define an unpleasant relationship between the nurse and others. This is sometimes the case with organ procurement practices. The physician, and in some cases the patient's family, may be angry about the requests placed upon them due to organ procurement policies. The nurse must struggle with the answers to angry demands as well as personal feelings about patient care. Policies and practices must be evaluated for their potential to support or obstruct nursing care and be modified if necessary.[9]

Finally, poor organization and poor management can contribute to work place stress. How long does it take to receive certain supplies? Are supplies and equipment adequate to meet demands? Is the lab adequately staffed to allow for quick responses to requests for emergency blood work? Are management directives clear? Is the patient acuity system accurate or is it outdated? Do staffing procedures lead to appropriate coverage? Assessing operations for strengths and weaknesses, and then changing ineffective processes will remove certain sources of stress. In the long run, increased productivity of the nursing department is sure to follow.

Several pertinent questions can be asked prior to the implementation of a new nursing structure. What are the present sources of stress? How high is the stress in the nursing environment? How do individuals respond to this stress? What will the introduction of a new structure do to the stress level?

Interventions to moderate stress are clear. The remediation of existent work place stressors, prompt conflict resolution during implementation, and the purposeful improvement of weak operations will help to assure that energies are directed towards change, rather than battling stressors.

DEALING WITH RESISTANCE

Avoiding Management by Hysteria

Hysteria develops in an organization when people panic about the personal consequences of an impending change. It is a highly contagious process that produces increased opposition to a new nursing structure. Managers begin to react to the hysteria rather than managing the change process. By understanding the sources of resistance to change, and strategies for reducing opposition, nursing leaders will avoid the trap of managing by hysteria.

Resistance can be defined as any behaviors that are aimed at keeping work behavior at the accepted norms of practice, instead of changing to meet new demands.[10] What people really oppose is not the technical change but the shifts in human relationships required by the new structure. In spite of the degree of participation in planning, the relationship aspect of any change must be managed in order to make sure that the change is accepted. For example, the implementation of shared governance structures requires a change in the relationship between managers and staff. It may also change the relationship of staff nurses to their manager.

In one organization, a new delivery system was erroneously rejected because of the social beliefs about how it would affect the relationships between staff nurses. In this example, the nurses grew increasingly concerned that their collegial relationships were being replaced with superior–subordinate relationships. Such a perception is laden with emotions. It can arise during the implementation of new nursing roles which appear to have "senior" and "junior" type role descriptions.

Implementation strategies must include information about not only how roles will change but also how they will remain the same. The environment must be scanned for misconceptions about how relationships will change under the new structure. Also, the introduction of a new structure must emphasize the equal contributions of all nurses to patient care. Nursing leaders must make sure that this attitude is shared by the entire nursing staff.

It is critical that potential changes be studied for their impact on social arrangements, both in sustaining them or threatening them. These relationships are not limited to peer relationships but extend to all of the interactions important to the individual nurse in the delivery of care. Some choices will have to be made. If the design of a new structure severely threatens existing social relationships, it will be as popular as a tax increase! A change in the design of the new structure will be necessary in order for implementation to proceed.[11]

Resistant behaviors can act as warning signals that hysteria and uncertainty are on the rise. Hysteria can be avoided by carefully examining implementation methods for their "people-friendliness." For example, it may be discovered that the knowledge of individuals affected by the change was not appropriately included during planning. This is a potential outcome if key groups do not participate in the planning process. Certain unpleasant consequences of implementation activities will not be identified early. Individuals and groups may be frustrated by the appearance of problems which they knew would occur, had anyone asked them.

Organizational demands for efficiency may be hurrying implementation. Certain system barriers may be overlooked. In such a scenario, nurses feel pushed and will inevitably push back.[12] Balancing demands for efficiency with time for learning is a major challenge during project implementation.

Sometimes the scrutiny of implementation activities reveals that attempts at participation to ensure commitment were not participative at all. Instead, the leaders used pseudoparticipative approaches to get people to do what was needed to be done.[13] For example, in one nursing organization, implementation was running smoothly in all but one clinical service. The manager had held several retreats outside of the hospital in order "to help nurses understand the change." To the outsider, this seemed to be an admirable approach, particularly in light of the resources expended to hold such sessions. Unfortunately, the sessions were orchestrated by the manager to pressure nurses into participation and to engender a view of the change that was compatible with the manager's perspective.

To the dismay of the project team, this clinical area displayed the most resistance to the change. These behaviors developed for several reasons. First, the manager did not clearly understand the new structure, but as a long-term manager he was afraid to admit his confusion and ask for help. This resulted in confusing and conflicting information being passed on to the staff. Second, opposition emerged because nurses saw the inherent dishonesty in his approach and felt manipulated. Had the nursing administrator insisted that the sessions be open to the project team and had even attended some of them herself, interventions could have been developed to reduce the sources of resistance.

Finally, opposition to a new nursing structure may emerge because of an overemphasis upon autonomy, empowerment, and professionalism rather than patient care.[14] These can be difficult and sometimes abstract concepts to translate to the bedside nurse. Autonomy may be experienced in the freedom of the nurse to act upon patient care needs without obstruction. Empowerment can mean a work place with no obstacles to patient care and easy access to the essential resources. Professionalism may simply mean the ability to accomplish nursing work without being stressed due to competing demands, inadequate staffing, low pay, or assuming the responsibilities of support staff.

This is not to say that autonomy, empowerment, and professionalism should not be the goals of a new nursing structure. However, in the early stages of change, all efforts must be made to translate these goals into the reality of nurses' everyday experiences.

PITFALLS IN CULTURE MANAGEMENT

Educational Errors

Selecting effective culture-changing activities is delicate and sensitive work. An area commonly overlooked is the role of the nursing educator in the introduction of change. If not managed appropriately, education errors will stimulate resistance and maintain the status quo.

Nurses move into education roles for many reasons. Some truly enjoy teaching. Others may simply be escaping the demands of the clinical nursing role. Some nurses may assume an educator role because it gives them more freedom and control over their work. These differences in motivation have a significant influence upon the accuracy with which an educator understands and communicates a new nursing structure.

Another source of difficulty can be found in the organizational structure of the education department itself. A centralized education department, reporting outside of the nursing organization, is an organizational structure that has a high potential for conflict from the competing needs of educators, the manager of the education department, and the nursing department.

For example, in one large organization, the administrator had decided that the education department needed to be down-sized. This decision was made at the same time that nursing had decided to implement a more participative organizational structure. It was believed that the two activities could occur in a parallel fashion, with the right preparation. However, the administrator of the education department was conflicted over having to deal with reduction of her department, feared a potential loss of status, and resented the nursing department's influence in the total organization. Consequently, this powerlessness and resentment was subtly conveyed to the education staff.

Since their loyalty was to the administrator and the whole organization, the nursing project was seen by educators as somehow responsible for their reduction in force. Unfortunately, the education department was expected to play a key role in the preparation of the nursing department for change. Had this been allowed to occur, their misperceptions of the change would certainly have been communicated to the nursing staff.

As a result, the introduction of the new nursing organizational structure was delayed several months. The resizing of the education department was completed and educators had renegotiated their roles within the nursing organization before implementation resumed.

Educators are in key positions to communicate and model the old behaviors which perpetuate the status quo instead of the behaviors required by the new nursing structures.[15]

Several strategies can be used to assure that educator role performance supports the restructuring project. Educators must accurately and completely understand the rationale for the change. They must be helped to describe the change in relation to organizational and nursing department goals, as well as the project implementation plan. If possible, educators should be included in the planning phase. The manager of the education department must be a key member of the project team. Because education errors may be very subtle, all educational materials should be examined for inadvertent presentations of old behaviors and modified, if warranted. For the same reason, presentations conducted by educators should be attended by selected project team members in order to facilitate the communication of accurate information.

Collusion

Collusion occurs when there is a silent agreement about the rules of interpersonal relationships and hidden agendas. These rules are always aimed at need satisfaction of some kind. Leaders and followers, in this instance, enter into an agreement to allow only a little change to occur. Such collusion develops when there are vague, unachievable, or incongruent goals. It is very unclear how the change will influence personal need satisfaction. Consequently, nurses are simply unable to integrate the change into their personal or professional need systems.

Some collusion can be limited by providing many informal opportunities to discuss the change. At this time, the nursing leader can clarify goals, identify incongruencies, and explain how the new structure will handle real differences in needs.[16] The clear delineation of which needs will be addressed will keep need satisfaction issues in the open, and will encourage the perception that needs are a legitimate topic of discussion.

Status and Personalities

Other relationship issues that must be managed during implementation include status problems, which make it difficult for managers and staff to act as partners in implementation. These difficulties are intensified when there are strong norms against partnerships. Limited support for mistakes, inadequate forums for discussion, and inadequate education about partnerships also contribute to status problems.

Finally, the personality of individual nurses may also stimulate opposition, particularly if they are in key implementation positions. A fear of being judged, fears of failure, inability to admit confusion, poor group skills, fierce independence, and certain personal beliefs are personality features that may produce resistant behaviors.[17] Direct supervision and coaching may help to alleviate these barriers to acceptance of the change. If not, the individual may need to consider leaving the organization or looking for a position not affected by the change.

MANAGING THE INTERPERSONAL NATURE OF CHANGE

A new structure will be successfully implemented through a series of decisions by individuals and groups, during which time the structure is either integrated into current practice or it is rejected.[18] The effective management of the organizational culture promotes acceptance of the new structure.

There are certain stages in the acceptance of a new nursing structure. In the *knowledge phase*, nurses are exposed to what the structure looks like, how it functions, and the benefits of change. In the persuasion stage, favorable or unfavorable attitudes are formed about the new structure. A decision is then made to accept or reject the new structure. If the new structure is accepted, the nurse begins to perform the expected behaviors. The *confirmation phase* signals the end of the *adoption phase*. The nurse is observed seeking reinforcement from others for the decision to change.[19]

The *persuasion phase* requires particular attention. Nurses are becoming more psychologically involved with the change. Through informal channels of communication, individuals acquire information about the new structure which will shape attitudes. In addition to formal education, implementation activities in this phase must include careful management of the informal communication system. How is the structure being perceived? Where are people going to get their information? Who are the sources of information? In these instances, what is being said about the structure is as important as who is saying it.[20] Certain individuals, who are part of the informal communication network, can undermine or promote acceptance of a new structure. Individuals in boundary-spanning roles, such as supervisors or clinical nurse specialists should be used to identify the information that exists within the informal communication system. Then methods can be applied which correct inaccurate information, provide missing information, and limit the influence of individuals who pass on bad information. These interventions strengthen the interpersonal network so that it can support the introduction of a new structure.

Recognizing the Importance of Networks

There are multiple communication networks in diverse and complex health care organizations. Nursing leaders must assure that an effective communication network is operational during the implementation of a major change. Networks of individuals and groups are interconnected through proximity, likeness of world view, and liaison communication forums. The acceptance of a change is partially determined by the effectiveness of these structures.[21]

In decentralized organizations, communication systems are spread across the nursing organization. Nurses, through their linkages with key cliques and access to information forums, experience significant influence over the implementation of a new structure. This strong communication network provides opportunities for nurses to identify which problems require immediate attention. As participants in strong networks, nurses will have a significant role in determining how the structure might be modified to better fit user needs.

However, decentralized communication structures can be problematic. If the change requires significant technical expertise, this skill cannot be easily spread through the communication structures. Furthermore, the nursing leader will find it very difficult to coordinate the flow, timing, and amount of information in the system.[22] In certain restructuring projects, it may be wise to develop a more centralized and more controlled system of communication. This is particularly true, for example, in the implementation of shared governance structures. Such a change is hard to communicate. It is difficult, at times, for nurses to understand the direction of the change. The implementation of shared governance is also a very complex change for any nursing organization to consider.

INTERVENING IN ROLE ISSUES

Effective nursing organizations function in an environment of information and communication instead of hierarchy. Members of the organization have the responsibility to make themselves understood, acquire the information needed to do their work, and provide adequate information to others.[23] Unfortunately, many nursing organizations are trapped in hierarchy. Fighting and intergroup conflict prevails because no one is sure of the information about the change. Some of the most important information concerns the delineation of effective nursing roles within the new nursing structure. As new nursing roles unfold, opportunities must be provided that help nurses to understand and perform new role behaviors. Also, information must be elicited from the new role incumbents about the adequacy of role definitions.

Two problems should be monitored for during the trial of new nursing roles. Consider the implementation of a new delivery system. *Role diffusion* may create threats to effective performance. This may occur when nursing activities are delegated or shared with other occupational groups possessing a narrower focus upon patient care.[24] Errors may be made when the abilities of such groups are overestimated, negatively influencing patient care. Role diffusion may be stressful to the nurse, depending upon the number of activities passed on to other groups. Patient care will become increasingly fragmented if role diffusion is extensive. Adequate time must be allowed for the testing of new roles. Also, monitoring for the presence of role diffusion will reduce the potential for such negative role outcomes.

Role expansion occurs when responsibilities are added to the nursing role.[25] Expanded accountabilities may produce confusion about performance priorities, boundary conflicts with other professionals, and role overload. New role occupants must be encouraged to discuss each of these potential problem areas and to recommend alternatives to role design.

MATCHING THE NEW STRUCTURE TO THE ENVIRONMENT

Nursing is at the heart of all patient care activities. Consequently, the strategies for completing the new nursing structure can have far-reaching implications for the nursing organization's influence and effectiveness within the larger organization. This premise is an important consideration when decisions are made about how a new structure will actually be constructed. Fifty percent of most decision-making difficulties encountered by organizations are the direct result of cumbersome or inadequate structures.[26] In order to prevent poor structure performance, nursing leaders must understand how certain structure features relate to the organizational environment. Successful structures will be designed and implemented based on an analysis of the new structure's centrality, flexibility, and ability to control resources.

Centrality

The centrality of a new nursing structure is reflected in the degree to which it is connected with the core activities of the nursing department and the whole health care organization.[27] For example, the introduction of a case management delivery system influences every activity of the health care organization. Simply put, nursing work flow is at the core of all of the activities within a health care organization. It touches every corner of the environment. The implementation of a new nursing structure must include a recognition of the influence that nursing work flow has upon the work of the rest of the organization.

If designed and executed appropriately, the structure enhances organizational performance and strengthens nursing's influence. If the structure performs poorly, the reverse is true. The nursing organization's influence is diminished and the goals of nursing lose support.

The central influence of a nursing structure are also diminished by the degree to which specialty demands are allowed to modify the structure features.[28] If there are multiple versions of the new structure in one organization, nursing work flow could be fragmented and not well understood by the rest of the organization. When determining the steps needed to complete a new structure, it is important to make sure that modifications are kept to a minimum.

Controlling Uncertainty

The delivery of patient care is not a predictable process. This fact is a crucial consideration in the execution of new nursing structures. Nursing structures must be designed to allow for the flexibility to meet unexpected occurrences in the environment and to gather resources at a moment's notice.[29]

Rules and guidelines for using the structure will necessarily accompany implementation. Care must be taken not to overspecify behaviors, thereby reducing flexibility. Nurses must be able to adjust the processes of the new structure so they can make decisions that limit or control uncertainty. Consequently, the authority of the nurse within the structure must be clearly identified. In large, complex organizations, this flexibility is essential in order for nurses to overcome the dual obstacles to the control of unpredictability: formalization and hierarchy.

Control Over Resources

The effectiveness and influence of a new nursing structure is also partially determined by its ability to enhance the control over resources. Resources are both observable and invisible. A new nursing structure must be enacted so that it easily accesses all categories of resources in the provision of patient care. Otherwise, the structure will be rejected due to poor performance. Inefficient resources hinder decision making because of inadequate access to critical resources.

Clearly, a structure must be composed so that all members of the nursing staff are able to participate fully. Implementation steps may add one group of staff at a time, until all key staff groups are integrated under the new system. If a particular group is struggling with performance under the new structure, its features should be examined to determine the source of the difficulty. Problems may be found to be due to knowledge/skill deficits of the group in question. However, it may be the structure itself that is impeding performance. If the latter is true, then the design of the structure should be modified to accommodate needs. Otherwise, the structure itself is a barrier to the achievement of quality care, because key nursing staff members are not able to perform well within it.

Access to the information needed to plan, organize, and perform quality patient care must be assured under the new structure. This important resource can be overlooked when deciding the arrangement of elements within a new nursing structure. Does the new design require new or different information than is currently available to nurses? What are the plans for acquiring access to this information? Does the new structure block access to critical information?

For example, in the implementation of product line management, access to the marketing and planning department's information may be a new information requirement for nurses acting as product line managers. Similarly, the implementation of case management requires some integration of medical and nursing information in the planning and coordination of care. If this integration does not exist, the structure may fail because of the lack of availability of integrated medical and nursing information. Before case management can be successfully introduced, medical staff relationships have to be assessed and decisions made about how to acquire critical patient care information.

A Fundamental Appreciation for Reality

The step-by-step introduction of a new nursing structure must be accompanied by a strong awareness of the realities of the environment. Patient care activities do not cease during implementation. The politics of the organization remain the same. A realistic transformation occurs with the application of certain important strategies. For example, a balance must be kept between moving too slow or too fast. While it is important to allow time for learning, too much time diminishes the urgency and momentum necessary for the political support of nursing goals.

As mentioned previously, care must be taken to avoid overloading the organization with too much change. The possibility of overload should be addressed in planning. However, unexpected demands for other kinds of change are bound to occur. The nursing leader must systematically evaluate the demands for additional change. Several pertinent questions can be asked:

1. What else is anticipated as changing during the time frame of implementation?
2. Will these other changes affect the nursing staff? How?
3. Will the scheduling of implementation activities take into consideration the other changes in the nursing or health care organization?
4. Are the unexpected changes absolutely necessary?
5. Can the nursing organization handle any more change? If not, which change will predominate?
6. Will implementation of the new structure need to be slowed down in order to accommodate emergent and necessary changes from unpredictable sources?

The project team can be of great assistance to the nursing leader in providing thoughtful answers to these difficult questions.

Another strategy for assuring that the implementation process is realistic is to allow for time-out from the change. The experience of change is exhausting. In order to avoid burnout and withdrawal from active participation in the change, nursing leaders can make sure that implementation steps include carefully planned time-out periods. During these times, small victories can be celebrated. Humor should be encouraged to help people let go of intensity. Retracing accomplishments will offset feelings of futility, because a structure is not up and running yet. Clearly, managing the pace of change, avoiding overload, allowing for time-outs, and celebrating victories will assure that new nursing structures are implemented with a realistic eye.

RE-EDUCATION STRATEGIES

Developing a Simple but Persuasive Message

The early preparation of the nursing environment is accomplished through education activities that carry the message about the new structure. If designed appropriately, education can delineate the need for the change and establish the belief that the new structure is a solution to the problem. Education methods range from formal in-services, formal/informal discussion groups, and published handbooks for new role incumbents. For example, some organizations have developed handbooks for staff participants on shared governance councils.

Rogers (1983) denotes several types of knowledge that are required for the acceptance of something new. All types of knowledge needs should be included in the design of education activities. *Awareness knowledge needs* include the requirement to understand that there is an urgent problem which requires resolution. The new structure needs to be accepted as a solution. *"How to" knowledge* is usually the focus for much of the education provided during a major change. This information provides guidelines to successful use of the structure and requisite behaviors, as well as the identification of formal sources of information regarding the change. *Theoretical knowledge* includes facts or principles about how the new structure works. This technical information is necessary for effective use of the new structure.[30]

An important goal in any education strategy is to reframe the new structure so that it is congruous with nurses' perceptions of reality. To reframe means to change the conceptual and/or emotional meanings of a certain experience and put it into another frame of reference.[31]

It is human nature to categorize or cluster meanings into groups determined by their meaning or value. This is what reality is to each individual. Certain experiences, such as expectations of the work place and related job performance, are placed into distinct categories of meaning. It is exceedingly difficult to change them. For example, reality to some nurses may be that "they" make decisions without considerations for the impact of such decisions upon nursing practice. The "we–they" dichotomy is believed to be the reality of the work place. When new participative structures are implemented, some nurses may reject them for being unrealistic. Education and experimenting with the change can introduce the notion that there are alternative realities. Then, definitions of reality become less rigid and more amenable to change.[32]

Education is particularly useful when it is conducted in advance of implementation and provided over time. If significant opposition to the change is anticipated then education should be introduced early. This is particularly true if the new structure is a radical departure from the present environment.[33] In the case described in Chapter 9, the implementation of product-line management was hindered by a failure to provide adequate education. Not enough time was allocated to education and the timing of the education was too late.

A series of educational sessions could be provided as the preliminary implementation activities in the introduction of a new nursing structure. Exhibit 4-1 provides a sample of how an education program might be designed in order to introduce case management.

Formalizing the Restructuring Project

What happens in the early days of implementation will influence the rest of the project. Nurse leaders must assure, by their words and their actions, that they take the implementation of the new structure seriously. There are several ways to formalize this support in the nursing environment. The top nursing executive should be present at all kick-off sessions. Later, milestone meetings should be held in order to convey the new vision and reinforce its value. This should never be left to subordinates. It is the top nursing leader who can truly convey both the excitement and the urgency associated with the change. Distinctive and carefully orchestrated meetings will create new rituals around the new nursing structures and help to allay fears.[34]

Exhibit 4-1 Nursing Discussion Group Topics for Sessions on Case Management

WEEK 1
- why a change is needed and why case management is the answer
- new work behaviors requiring adjustment
- definition of case management
- formal and informal rules
- workload specification
- forums for communication

WEEK 2
- managed care vs. case management
- divisions of labor: case managers and associates
- the role of support staff/nursing
- the role of support staff/non-nursing
- mechanisms for integrating patient care
- overcoming tradition
- delegation skills
- testing new behaviors
- resource identification

WEEK 3
- case management values
- individual differences—functional vs. nonfunctional
- conflict resolution approaches
- opportunities for evaluating the system
- deadlines for role acquisition
- financial procedures

WEEK 4
- case management in relation to nursing organization goals
- case management in relation to health care organization goals
- benefits to individuals, groups, and the organization
- implementation time lines
- evaluation methods
- coping with confusion
- options available for individuals

Another tangible indicator of the importance of the project is the establishment of a project room. The assignment of physical space to a project cannot be underestimated. For example, in one organization, a physical representation of the change occurred quite by accident. It served to formalize a new order within the nursing department. A confidential method was needed to collect evaluation surveys from the nursing staff during the implementation of a shared governance structure. It was decided that facilities management would build wooden "shared governance" letter boxes and put them in the conference rooms of each nursing unit, so that staff could anonymously return questionnaires. These boxes eventually were used for communications between the participative councils and the nursing units. They became the symbols of the council structure on each nursing unit. Since shift report was often held in conference rooms, the boxes served to remind staff of the organizational commitment to the new council structure.

A project room should include a desk, a telephone, and the assignment of clerical support for project participants, particularly staff nurses. Project and planning team meetings could be held in the project room, since most of the documents pertaining to the change would be housed in files kept in this room. Schedules of the implementation and tracking information could be posted on the walls. A library of relevant materials could be available for check-out or copying. Clearly, a project room would embody the seriousness of the commitment to change.[35]

Another method for indicating the priority of a project is to assign a formal logo and/or a value statement to all communication about the change. This approach not only emphasizes the importance of the change but also serves as a constant reminder, ultimately raising awareness.[36]

MENTAL OBSTACLES: MAJOR BARRIER TO SUCCESS

Cultural activities are not limited to the early phases of the change. Commitment is continually evaluated, accompanied by the constant reinforcement of expectations.

For example, in the implementation of product-line management, the nursing leader must periodically attend multidisciplinary staff meetings to reinforce the role, authority, and importance of professional groups. The change must be re-enforced by constant communication of the urgency and the excitement accompanying product-line management. The nursing leader must communicate the vision not only with formal dialogue but with active listening, a strong presence, and promises kept.[37]

QUESTIONS TO GUIDE ENVIRONMENTAL STRATEGY DEVELOPMENT

1. Which features of the nursing organization's culture will promote or obstruct the implementation of new nursing structures? How will obstructing features be ameliorated?
2. How does the culture of the whole health care organization compare to that of the nursing culture? Are the gaps problematic for successful implementation? How will these gaps be addressed?
3. What stressors exist in the present nursing environment? How are they experienced by individuals and groups? How will these stressors be modified prior to implementation?
4. How will work relationships be altered or sustained as the result of the new nursing structure? Can the structure be modified so as to lessen the degree of change in social relationships?
5. Who are the key players in the informal communication network? How will this network be monitored for commitment and accuracy of information?
6. What communication structure exists presently in the organization? Is it sufficient to carry the information needed for the change?
7. Are nursing roles clearly defined, with time lines for the formalization of new nursing role behaviors?
8. Are there role diffusion and role expansion problems? How will these influence the implementation of new nursing structures?
9. How does the new structure match the organizational environment? Is it flexible, central to the work of nursing and controlling of resources?
10. Is the change process being facilitated in a realistic manner?
11. Does the education of key groups address awareness, "how to," and theoretical knowledge?
12. Do the formal and informal opportunities for education include the reframing of reality, to include the new structure as an alternative to encountered difficulties?

13. What methods will be employed to formalize the restructuring project?

NOTES

1. Rogers, E. (1983). *The Diffusion of Innovation*. New York: The Free Press, p. 163.
2. Deal, T.E. and Kennedy, A.A. (1982). *Corporate Cultures*. Reading, MA: Addison-Wesley Publishing Company, Inc.
3. Munroe, D.J. (1988). Commitment of part-time nursing personnel: A challenge. *Nursing Management,* 19(12), 59–61.
4. Cook, R.A. and Lafferty, J.L. (1989). *Level V: Organizational Culture Inventory*. Plymouth, MI: Human Synergistics, 1987, 1989.
5. Cooke, R.A. and Rousseau, D.M. (1988). Behavioral norms and approach to organizational cultures. *Group and Organizational Studies,* 13(3), 245–273 (1989).
6. Cook, R.A. and Lafferty, J.L. (1989).
7. Wadsworth, N.S. (1986). Managing organizational stress in nursing. *Journal of Nursing Administration,* 16(2), 21–28.
8. Maslach, C. (1982). *Burnout—The Cost of Caring*. New York: Prentice-Hall, Inc.
9. Ibid., pp. 29–51.
10. Rogers, E. (1983), p. 163.
11. Lawrence, P.R. (1988). How to deal with resistance to change. *People: Managing Your Most Important Asset*. Boston, MA: Harvard Business Review Press, pp. 41–43.
12. Ibid., p. 42.
13. Ibid., pp. 36–44.
14. Bocchino, C.A. (1991). An interview with Joyce C. Clifford. *Nursing Economics,* 9(1), p. 8.
15. Goren, B. and O'Howay, R. (1985). Why health care teams do not change. *Journal of Nursing Administration,* 15(7), pp. 9–16.
16. Ibid., pp. 13–16.
17. Zaltman, G. and Duncan, R. (1977). *Strategies For Planned Change*. New York: John Wiley and Sons, pp. 86–89.
18. Rogers, E. (1983), p. 163.
19. Ibid., p. 164.
20. Ibid., pp. 169–172.
21. Ibid., pp. 272–280.
22. Ibid., pp. 294–337.
23. Drucker, P.F. (1990). *Managing The Nonprofit Organization*. New York: Harper Collins Publishers, p. 115.

24. Singleton, E.K. and Nael, F.C. (1984). Role clarification: A pre-requisite to autonomy. *Journal of Nursing Administration,* 15(10), 17–22.
25. Ibid., p. 19.
26. Peters, T. (1990). Flawed company structures hurt the decision-making process. Comment section. *The Business Journal,* November 5, Phoenix, Arizona.
27. Holzel, C.B. (1989). Using Structural Power Sources To Increase Influence. *Journal of Nursing Administration,* 19(11), 10–14.
28. Ibid., pp. 10–11.
29. Ibid., p. 14.
30. Rogers, E. (1983), pp. 167–168.
31. Watzdawick, P., Weakland, J., and Fisch, R. (1974). *Change.* New York: W.W. Norton Publishing, pp. 95–98.
32. Ibid., pp. 97–98.
33. Zaltman, G. and Duncan, R. (1977), pp. 110–112.
34. Waterman, R.H. (1990). *Advocacy: The Power To Change.* San Francisco: Whittle Direct Books, pp. 31–53.
35. Ibid., p. 46.
36. Ibid., p. 50.
37. Moss Kanter, R. (1989). *When Giants Learn To Dance.* New York: Simon and Schuster, pp. 82–89.

CHAPTER 5

Matching New Visions to Reality: Restructuring Demands and the Nursing Management Team

No major change should be considered without a careful examination of the beliefs, knowledge, and technical skills of each member of the nursing management team. Deficiencies in management expertise lay at the heart of many failed projects. The manager must keep operations running smoothly during the turbulent times of transition to a new structure. Managers also intervene in the personal experience of change, by translating the goals of the project into the performance of subordinates. The ability to manage change, while also assuring the effectiveness of everyday operations, is the ultimate test of manager expertise.

This chapter addresses those core competencies of managers believed to be central during a restructuring project. Decision-making abilities, people skills, integration expertise, political knowledge, and motivational abilities are discussed in detail.

Managers themselves may be the single biggest obstacle to the accomplishment of a successful change. Why? The project planning team often overlooks the needs of managers during times of transition. The focus of much of the planning and implementation activities is on the needs and concerns of the staff and not the managers. What follows can be manager opposition to the change. A new structure can intensify manager job security fears. Managers may be expected to take on the implementation of a new structure with no relief from other duties. Management roles may be inadequately defined. There may be no safe place for managers to question the change. Competition in the manager group may contribute to fragmentation of efforts.

The top nursing administrator is in a key position to intervene on behalf of managers who struggle with new performance expectations during a major change. Expectations must be established that undermining behavior should be dealt with quickly and directly. Hospital administrators must be kept informed of the status of the change, including resource needs. A strong management development program must be supported.

If the needs of managers are not addressed during the implementation phase, the potential for negative outcomes is quite high. The result may be poorly performing structures and dysfunctional operations. Staff dissatisfaction will intensify and the credibility of nursing goals within the larger organization will be lost.

DECISION-MAKING SKILLS

Johnson (1990) argues that management decision making is the core component of nursing management activities. Decision-making effectiveness is determined by the assumptions held by the manager, including:

1. basic beliefs about nursing, the patient, and the organization
2. personal and professional ideals
3. nursing knowledge
4. management knowledge
5. personal/professional values.

The manner in which a problem is identified, the solution selected from the problem resolution stage, and the behaviors engaged in to implement solutions are more related to the manager's world view than technical skill.[1]

Difficulties in the project implementation phase arise when managers lack technical skills, and when their world view does not match with the world view required for support of the new structure. For example, necessary organizational integration activities may be overlooked because the manager holds a strong nursing ideal of loyalty to nursing, instead of a systems viewpoint. Similarly, the flexibility necessary for effective planning may be limited because of a belief that the nursing department has a predetermined plan. Efficiency may be valued over innovation and creativity, so that time is not allowed for the necessary problem solving during implementation.[2]

The most successful world view for nursing managers is a systems viewpoint. It allows for decision making to occur as events unfold in the internal and external environment. The implementation of a new nursing structure is thought of in terms of how it affects all parts of the system. Nursing managers believe that they have a key role in the facilitation of the system, not just the new nursing structure. The systems viewpoint also promotes participation, because key individuals and groups are thought of as important system components.

Effective management skills are both tangible and intangible. In assessing the expertise of the management group, both categories must be considered. Some skills can be assessed through direct observation. Others can only be examined by listening to subordinates and sensing needs in the environment. Exhibit 5-1 summarizes the tangible and intangible skills of nursing managers.

PEOPLE SKILLS

Effective management outcomes are essential for the successful implementation of new nursing structures. The nursing management

Exhibit 5-1 Tangible and Intangible Skills of Nurse Managers

Tangible Skills	*Intangible Skills*
• planning	• beliefs
• organizing	• values
• controlling	• ideals
• directing	• decision making
• evaluating	• judgment
• systems viewpoint	• integrating skills
• human management skills	• political savvy
• flexibility/negotiation/compromise	• analytic thinking
• health/nursing knowledge	• vision
• financial skills	

team is responsible for the people performance which is essential to the organization's capacity to succeed. By virtue of their relationship to the professional staff, the managers are able to translate the goals of the organization into the activities of subunits within the nursing organization. People skills include communication, negotiation, group facilitation, promotion of trust, and excellent listening skills.

Successful nursing managers have strong abilities in learning about, interpreting, and implementing organizational objectives.[3] These skills are then readily transferred to the facilitation of change within individuals and groups. How are implementation goals introduced in the manager's area of responsibility? Is it an open process or limited to a select few? How are the goals of the new nursing structure communicated to the nursing staff? An open goal-setting process provides nurses many opportunities for input. This kind of communication will develop strong links between organizational goals and nursing staff performance. Ideas will not disappear for lack of anything to hang them on.

Is the manager's budget tied to the operational goals? Does the budget cycle follow the establishment of annual goals? When this relationship exists, it is likely that goals are realistic. The challenges faced by the organization in goal achievement will be more clearly described for all concerned.

Does the manager spend time analyzing the goals of subordinates in relation to the goals of the nursing organization? Are regular meetings scheduled with individual staff to promote goal achievement? Are management meetings effective? Does the top nursing administrator attend staff meetings periodically to communicate the vision and the status of nursing organization goals?

The ability to help an organization through a major change is a requisite skill for nursing managers at all levels during the implementation phase. People skills may take precedent, at times, over technical skills. In a recent study of middle manager effectiveness, researchers discovered that human management skills were rated as the most important, followed by the ability to be flexible, and the presence of negotiating/compromise skills. Financial expertise was not at the top of the list, despite the economics of the health care environment. This was attributed to a possible increase in comfort with finance, which managers had to develop in response to environmental demands.[4]

Successful managers of people see themselves as leaders and change agents. They are accountable for mentoring, facilitating institutional goals through staff performance, and helping staff to both cope with and accept a new nursing structure.[5]

If nursing leaders recognize the personal nature of change, then certain change activities will predominate. Change is considered as a personal skill-building experience. Training allows enough time for the change to take hold. The project is not overmanaged. Allowances are made for modification based on individual and group feedback. This trims the new structure to better fit with the existing culture. Identified heros are placed in key positions during implementation. This allows for the mentoring and role-modeling of appropriate new behaviors.[6]

Care is taken to assure that significant relationships among individuals, groups, and nursing work units are not unduly disturbed. Regularly scheduled discussion sessions build trust, give nurses the necessary time to integrate feelings and awareness of the need for change, and will identify additional supports and resources.[7]

INTEGRATION SKILLS AND FUNCTIONS

During the implementation phase, the integration functions of the nurse manager are of paramount importance. These include the ability to recognize and modify deficiencies of a new structure in relation to both stated goals and operations. Managers must continually scan the organization for the "goodness-of-fit" of the nursing structure. This requires a pro-active mind set. By monitoring the outcomes of implementation activities, managers are positioned to design new and better nursing structures and processes. Tension and stress are redirected toward problem solving.[8]

As the primary link to the professional staff, the nursing manager is responsible for integrating the visions of the new structure performance with the reality of the work place demands. During the implementation phase, the nursing manager becomes the symbol for the new order. If nursing managers are confused, threatened by change, or uninformed about the implementation plan, then the manager-as-symbol process will convey the same messages to subordinates. Important feedback about structure performance will be missed.

Another integrating function of the manager assumes great importance during times of transition. This function is found in the activities that regulate the uncertainty coming from the change. Nursing managers buffer the patient care environment so that patient care is not adversely influenced.[9] A good manager scrutinizes the environment to determine where the gaps are between people and the environment, including the new nursing structure. The quality of patient care and the degree of stress experienced by the nursing staff during a major change are clear indicators of the manager's ability to "supervise the seams between people and the environment."[10] By focusing upon the uncertainty of the environment, the nursing manager helps the staff to integrate the change, while delivering quality care.

POLITICAL SKILLS

"Being political" is a characteristic often rejected by nurses. Somehow the word "politics" conjures up values that seem to be in opposition to the traditional nursing values of caring. Yet, the ability to integrate the vision of new nursing structures with the reality of the environment is directly related to the political acumen of nursing managers.

Political skills can be roughly grouped into the following sets of activities:[11]

1. Pro-actively seeking opportunities to demonstrate the values of nursing work to the outcomes of the whole organization
2. Providing for the comfort of subordinates through planning to promote predictability but preparing staff for the fact that plans do (and must) change as demands change
3. Continually re-evaluating priorities to assure they match the priorities of the organization
4. Being open to change by identifying the right issues at the right time by accurately reading the culture
5. Being adept at selling others on oneself and persuading people to accept ideas and solutions
6. Avoiding reliance upon unchallenged authority to accomplish change but encourage participation
7. Skillfully developing and participating in work teams
8. Being comfortable in sharing power through collaboration, negotiation, and partnerships.

DEVELOPING EFFECTIVE REWARD SYSTEMS

Another valuable skill during implementation is the manager's expertise in rewarding innovation, creativity, and problem solving during the introduction of change. The achievement of a well integrated and successfully performing nursing structure requires the creative talents of many individuals.[12]

During implementation, most nurses seek information about what behaviors will be rewarded. They then look for opportunities to perform these behaviors. In most nursing organizations, performance reviews and career ladders function as defined reward systems. Once a new nursing structure has been completed, it is formalized in these activities. However, career ladders are limited in that they only reward behavior that can be objectively defined.

How can creativity be stimulated and then rewarded? First, the nursing manager must strive to minimize the intensity associated with the change. This means that the new structure is discussed in a relaxed and informal atmosphere. Individuals are encouraged to think about the possibility of changing things, if necessary. The implementation plan must be seen as somewhat fluid, rather than as something with a life of its own. The manager can ask everyone to identify a question about the implementation, in order to stimulate problem solving. Finally, mistakes must be viewed as learning opportunities. Rarely are solutions perfect the first time around. By communicating an open mind about failure, the manager will stimulate and reward the necessary experimentation leading to effective nursing structures.

Nurses work for a variety of reasons. There is often not one singularity of purpose within the nursing staff of most nursing organizations. What is satisfying to one nurse may be of no interest to another, depending upon where the individual is in relation to the nursing work cycle. However, nurses do agree that nursing work should be intellectually stimulating, pay should be commensurate with work, and nurses should be recognized as professionals.[13]

How can reward systems be designed to meet these multiple needs? One strategy is to introduce select work place changes along with the new nursing structure. In this way, change is linked with a tangible benefit for all nurses. For example, an alternative organizational structure may be introduced along with new nursing shifts or improved pay practices.[14] Structures that increase participation and control over nursing practice can be introduced with additional resources, such as the unit personnel described in Chapter 8.

Some errors in rewarding new behaviors can occur. The manager may unknowingly reward some behaviors more than others. The wrong behaviors may be rewarded due to confusion about the change or hidden agendas. The manager may focus on what is good rather than what is necessary.[15] Nursing managers must be careful that value judgments do not cloud the manner in which they reward new nursing behaviors.

COUNTERACTING MANAGER RESISTANCE

Rarely is manager resistance to a new structure readily observable. Managers are often the veterans of many organizational changes and believe that their success is tied to the public support of a new order.

OVERLOOKED NEEDS

Why would nursing managers fail to support a new structure? The new structure may be incongruent with their predominant management style, particularly in the implementation of participative structures. More likely, the needs of managers during transitions have simply been overlooked by the project team.[16] In one organization, the design and implementation of a participative nursing organizational structure did not include nurse managers on any committees concerned with clinical practice. This decision not only heightened manager suspicion and distrust, but resulted in missed opportunities for managers to understand staff nurse needs. Some individuals over-reacted to the artificial division of clinical and management decisions, by refusing to participate in *any* clinical decision making.

An alternative approach in this case is to encourage management participation in the early phases of implementation, with a clearly stated timetable for transition to clinical staff leadership.

Clearly, managers must have access to both the information and the experiences that will advance their understanding of the new structure. This is the only way they can facilitate the commitment and participation of others.

JOB SECURITY ISSUES

Job security issues are always part of the project implementation phase. However, if the new structure has the potential for reducing management positions, these fears will be intensified. The power of job insecurity to slow down implementation was observed in a nursing organization implementing case management. Nursing managers became frightened when they read an article that referenced a case management as a partial response to vacant manager positions. Several sessions needed to be held with the manager group to address perceptions of case management as a covert strategy to eliminate management positions. Even then, distrust lingered in the management group.

TOO MANY DEMANDS

Unwillingness to change may arise if the additional work of implementation is added to current management duties without relief. How are the nursing management roles designed? Too many performance demands result in exhaustion and the withdrawal of managers from involvement in the organization. This clearly jeopardizes the facilitation of implementation activities.[17] Manager responsibilities should be monitored for the presence of too many demands, to the neglect of implementation activities. Some managers may need assistance to delegate certain functions to assistant managers. Other managers will need assigned support staff, to ease some of the added responsibilities during implementation.

INADEQUATE ROLE DEFINITIONS

Do management roles allow the necessary judgment and authority for work schedules, designing and implementing new processes to improve patient care, or other decisions?[18] If managers themselves are not fully empowered to manage, then they will find it exceedingly difficult to manage the turbulence of change. This difficulty can be mistaken as resistance, when management roles themselves are the obstacles to successful change.

Managers may also resist the reordering of things because of inadequate role clarification. This occurs when the nursing administrator does not communicate and model the new management skills and behaviors. Managers become unclear about what they are supposed to do differently under the new structure, and worry about changes in the evaluation of their work.

A LACK OF SUPPORT FORUMS

A lack of forums for expressing disagreement may also hinder the change project. Inflexible meeting agendas and the lack of networking groups leave little room for disagreement and send it underground. This is particularly true when disagreement about the new structure is considered by the top nursing administrator as unprofessional or lacking in vision.

Support forums are effective to the degree that competition in the manager group is at a minimum. Competition between managers arises when it is perceived that there are limited opportunities for advancement in the organization. Inadequate compensation and lack of recognition for contribution may also stimulate competition in the management group.[19]

Support networks should be encouraged for the nursing management group. However, it is essential that such networks do not allow in the expression of concerns without action. This results in the isolation of important concerns from issues identified in the larger organization. Subgroup issues are not recognized and continue to intensify because they are not addressed by the project team.

Nursing managers must be held accountable for taking their concerns to those in a position to do something about them. If the discomfort in publicly voicing concerns is impeding implementation, a liaison manager could be temporarily appointed to the project team. This individual has clearly defined responsibilities to bring management group concerns to the appropriate decision-making bodies, until trust is established.

DYSFUNCTIONAL MANAGER PERFORMANCE

Dysfunctional manager role implementation will continue as long as the manager's supervisor allows it to flourish. Supervisors of managers must accept the discomforting information that one of their subordinates is undermining the restructuring project. These issues must be dealt with immediately through the direct supervision of resistant individuals. Unfortunately, some supervisors simply fail to intervene in undermining behaviors. On the other hand, they may intervene only after considerable damage has been done. A certain loyalty to long-term subordinates, a strong tendency to avoid conflict, or a concern about the resistant manager's influence in the system may result in avoidance behavior.

Administrative avoidance behaviors are sometimes expressed by making an inappropriate decision to wait for peer pressure to produce the required behaviors in an undermining individual. Significant damage to the implementation process can occur while waiting. Another avoidance strategy is to rationalize the undermining manager's behaviors by attributing them to other stressors. Finally, avoidance may be expressed by simply looking the other way. The net effect is to send a strong message that top management support for the project is inconsistent or missing altogether. What follows is a hesitancy on the part of individual managers to take the risks necessary for successful implementation. The management group will experience increased confusion about the direction of the change.

It is imperative that resistant manager behaviors be addressed during the project implementation phase so that they do not stimulate further resistance within the nursing organization. However, dealing with resistance must be balanced with giving people enough time to learn new behaviors.

The role of the nursing administrator in relation to individual managers and the nursing management team is crucial for successful implementation. In addition to providing clear role expectations, direct supervision, and personal coaching, those individuals who supervise the manager must also assure that people are not placed in positions that are beyond their skill level. Sometimes certain managers, by virtue of their position, are assigned to facilitate a set of implementation activities. However, these individuals may lack the expertise to succeed. This is not only personally devastating to the individual but also harms the introduction of change. Leadership positions during implementation should simply be assigned by skill rather than by position. Assignments need to be accompanied by a valuing attitude that conveys the message that everyone has something to contribute.

THE POWER OF A SINGULAR VOICE FOR NURSING

Translating the needs of nursing to the next level is an obvious and necessary nursing management skill. However, this critical function may be lost, depending upon the design of the top nursing administrator role. New role definitions for top nursing administrators are widening in scope to include responsibility for the other patient care services provided in the health care organization.[20] This broader sphere of influence promotes the coordination of patient care activities, but may present unique challenges in the implementation phase of restructuring projects. The tangible translation of nursing goals, needs, and concerns can be significantly diminished because of the competing need of a broader world view within the same administrative role.

Nevertheless, the implementation of new nursing structures requires that *someone* have the accountability for translating to the administrative staff the reason for turbulence in the system and for identifying those organizational resources necessary for success. Without these initiatives, top administrative support for the project could be withdrawn due to unfounded concerns about the change or misperceptions from inadequate information.

Significant implementation errors may not be recognized by the top nursing administrator with an expanded responsibility. Traditional nurse executive responsibilities for nursing department management are commonly delegated to those individuals who manage the core clinical nursing departments. This may make the accurate identification and trending of implementation problems quite difficult.[21] The extent to which the nursing leader is able to solve these problems will determine the degree to which the health care organization tolerates the turbulence attributed to the changes. If this important translation fails, the project will be placed in considerable jeopardy.

Some organizations have addressed the translation and role diffusion problems of expanded top nursing administration roles by appointing a director of nursing. This person acts as the spokesperson and deals with the coordination issues posed by the decentralization of nursing organizations.[22] This approach will succeed to the extent that the addition of a management layer is truly supported both within and outside of the nursing organization. It may be very difficult to justify the need for such a position in the current fiscal environment. Another solution may be to include key health care administrators as members of the project team. Also, middle managers in the nursing organization must have the freedom to determine changes in implementation activities as well as the accountability for successful nursing structures.

MANAGEMENT DEVELOPMENT NEEDS

Ideally, a strong management development program should precede or, if necessary, accompany the implementation of major change. In this manner, managers are given the opportunity to integrate the change into their role performance and develop the requisite skills for successful implementation activities.

The content of such a program is illustrated in Exhibit 5-2. These areas can be developed through formal education sessions, self-study/self-assessment, continuing education, or formal classroom work and personal coaching.

In summary, the following strategies will support nursing manager effectiveness in the introduction and facilitation of successful new nursing structures:

- Assure manager access to adequate information about the impending change through participation in planning, formal/informal education, and experimentation in safe situations.
- If management positions will be eliminated, be honest about it. Counsel/coach affected individual for positive transition to new roles.
- Design management roles with the three A's: authority, accountability, and appropriate expectations.
- Provide forums for discussion.
- Directly confront undermining behavior. Do not give into the temptation to wait it out. Provide resources for learning but set realistic deadlines for the appearance of supportive behaviors.
- Assess the management team for technical skills. Provide intensive education to correct deficiencies. Recruit new talent if necessary.
- Provide a substantial management development program prior to initiating the new structure so that nursing managers are well prepared to facilitate the change.

Exhibit 5-2 Management Development Content for the Introduction of New Nursing Structures

Structure Information

- relationship to organizational mission
- relationship to past changes
- concept of new structure
- terms and definitions—relationship to past changes
- implementation plans and schedules
- resources
- expected outcomes

Role Information

- behaviors expected to facilitate change
- new responsibilities demanded by the new structure and time lines for acquisition
- self-assessment of technical skills and personal development plan
- manager relationships to planning and project teams
- the nature of change

Human Management Skills

- motivation theories
- conflict management
- participation
- group facilitation skills
- dealing with resistant or undermining behaviors
- integrating skills

Personal Issues

- personal/professional beliefs, values, ideals, and knowledge and their relationship to the vision and the goals of the new structure
- time management
- delegation
- stress management
- management skill assessment

QUESTIONS TO GUIDE MANAGEMENT DEVELOPMENT

1. What are the beliefs, knowledge, values, ideals, and technical skills of the nursing management team?
2. Can discrepancies between the world view of managers and the viewpoint required for a new structure be detected?
3. What are the people skills of the management team? How are these demonstrated within areas of responsibility? How do subordinates describe their manager?
4. How are managers integrating the new structure into their present operations?
5. Is the management team politically savvy?
6. How do managers typically reward performance?
7. Do formal reward systems meet the needs of the new structure? If not, what is being done to change them?
8. How does the management team perceive the change?
9. Is the nursing organization structured for the effective coordination of the change? Are managers' roles designed well?
10. Do managers have the resources necessary to both direct operations and facilitate the change?
11. Does the new structure eliminate manager positions? How is this being handled?
12. Do managers have a safe place to express their concerns?
13. Is dysfunctional behavior addressed effectively by the supervisors of managers?
14. Is there one voice for nursing? If not, who is communicating the status of the change, interpreting turbulence, and identifying resource requirements to the health care organization's administrator?

NOTES

1. Johnson, L.J. (1990). The influence of assumptions on effective decision-making. *Journal of Nursing Administration,* 18(12), 23–27.
2. Ibid., p. 25.
3. Christen, J. (1988). The changing nature of first-line supervision. *The Health Care Supervisor,* 5(2), 34–36.

4. Patz, J.M., Biordi, D.L., and Hom, K. (1991). Middle manager nurse effectiveness. *Journal of Nursing Administration,* 21(1), 15–24.
5. Flarey, D. (1991). Redesigning management roles. *Journal of Nursing Administration,* 21(2), 40–50.
6. Deal, T.E. and Kennedy, A.A. (1982). *Corporate Cultures.* Reading, MA: Addison-Wesley Publishing Company, pp. 164–169.
7. Barnes, A.K., Harmon, P., and Kisch, J.P. (1986). A displacement orientation program. *Journal of Nursing Administration,* 16(7), 46–56.
8. Katz, R.L. (1974). Skills of an effective administrator. *Harvard Business Review,* 62(7), 91–92.
9. Gilmore, T.N. (1990). Effective leadership during organizational transition. *Nursing Economics,* 8(3), 135–141.
10. Ibid., p. 138.
11. Moss Kanter, R. (1981). *The Meaning of "Influence Skills" in Today's New Corporation.* Cambridge, MA: Good Measure, Inc., pp. 59–63.
12. Rogers, E. (1983). *The Diffusion of Innovation.* New York: The Free Press, p. 219.
13. Smeltzer, C. (1990). The Chicago Plan: Innovative strategies to change nurses' work patterns. *Journal of Nursing Administration,* 20(11), 3–6.
14. *The Changing American Work Place: Work Alternative in the 80's.* An American Management Association Report. New York: American Management Association, 1985, pp. 17–19.
15. Kerr, S. (1974). On the folly of rewarding A while hoping for B. *Academy of Management Journal,* 18(4), pp. 61–74.
16. Lawrence, P.R. (1988). How to deal with resistance to change. *People: Managing Your Most Important Asset.* Boston, MA: Harvard Business Review Press, p. 41.
17. Ibid., pp. 59–63.
18. Klein, J.A. (1984). Why supervisors resist employee involvement. *Howard Business Review,* 62(7), 87–95.
19. Ibid., p. 90.
20. Singleton, E.K. and Comeron, F. (1988). Nursing leadership: The effects of organizational structure. *Journal of Nursing Administration,* 18(10), 10–14.
21. Ibid., pp. 10–11.
22. Ibid., p. 13.

CHAPTER 6

Implementing a Product Line Management Structure in a Rehabilitation Hospital

Rhonda M. Anderson

Health care in the United States has experienced many difficult times and changes. These rapid changes, without fully planned and executed responses, have caused chaos in much of the health care industry. The history of these changes is the foundation necessary to understand the needed changes of today and to assure future changes are better designed and implemented.

HISTORICAL OVERVIEW

From the 1960s to the 1980s, most citizens who had some type of health care coverage had it through a private insurance company. Middle America received the health care coverage through their employers. Governmental monies were available to expand the supply of physicians and to rapidly improve and increase technology. A philosophy of removing all barriers to access of health care was ascribed to in the 1960s. Medicare and Medicaid were available to expand the supply of physicians and to rapidly improve and increase technology. The elderly thought they would be cared for for life because they had Medicare coverage. Hospitals were paid by the indemnity plans at approximately 80% of charges. Medicare paid on the basis of a hospital's costs plus some overhead and depreciation costs. Capital dollars for technology and physical plant expansion were extremely easy to acquire. During this era, there was a movement to massively transfuse the health care system. The philosophy during this time was that all persons had a right to health care and they would be taken care of regardless of ability to pay.

In the early 1970s, big businesses started to be concerned because the cost of their insurance premiums had consumed a large percentage of their profits. Citizens continued to use the doctor and hospital for every little physical ailment, enjoying health care as their birthright.

These behaviors continued to increase health care costs. With this overuse also came a more litigious society. Malpractice premiums grew at exponential rates. Citizens' mentality was not to own their responsibility in the wellness–illness continuum. Their life-styles reflected a need to overindulge without regard for their health.

During this 20-year period, hospitals faced many changes. In the first ten years rapid hospital and program growth occurred. Various types of specialized hospital departments developed. Most of these departments could charge for their services or products and the hospital was compensated by a third-party payor. The hospital departments were very functional and independent in the care rendered and in their charge structure. Nursing departments flourished in the same way. They grew and became more specialized. Nursing care was not a line item charge on the patient's bill, but was considered a part of the room rate. In most institutions, a department could add staff if they linked it to the revenue they could produce. For nursing, this was more difficult because they were considered cost producers, not revenue producers. However, full-time equivalents per occupied bed began to increase.

In the next ten-year period, "cost containment" were the buzz words. A major problem began to develop for hospitals in this scenario because the consumers of goods and services still wanted all their health care needs paid for and access to the health care system whenever they felt it necessary. This demand was inevitable, since no one in the country developed or implemented a change in the philosophy of the health care system. Technology continued to improve and every hospital wanted the newest and best equipment. The thought was that the best high technology environment would draw physicians and patients to the facility. Nursing was trying to establish their role as revenue producers, not just expense to the hospital. There was a move to separate nursing charges from the room rate and develop a line item on the patient bill for nursing care. This was just beginning to happen when major, unplanned changes in reimbursement took place.

In spite of pleas and strategies to decrease health care costs, the costs continued to rise. In the early 1980s the United States averaged $360 per day per patient and $3,450 per admission. This was higher than Japan, Canada, the United Kingdom, France, or Germany.[1] The government was very concerned because the Medicare trust fund funds were projected to be fully consumed by 1985. The percent of the gross national product spent on health care was 11% by the mid 1980s.

Technology poured into the health care facilities and caused devastation. The human resources developed in the 1960s and 1970s were also pouring into the health care industry and causing an oversupply.

Obviously something had to be done, and it was. The problem, however, escalated because only one part of the industry changed—reimbursement. The rest of the system had no planned response to this change. The federal government determined they would pay a preset price for a patient's hospitalization by diagnosis. Managed care plans were developed by businesses. This concept involved a monthly prepayment by employees for their health care. Health maintenance organizations and other managed health care programs entered the arena. These types of programs required a change of attitude and behavior on the part of the consumer and provider. Neither the consumer nor the provider was prepared for or understood this new philosophy. The consumer could join one of the managed care programs. Consumers paid a set monthly fee and received all their health care from that program. Physicians in those programs were compensated in a variety of ways, generally not on a fee for service basis as they had been under previous reimbursement. The specialists were contained in this scheme because consumers could not self-refer.

The "gatekeeper" concept developed where a primary care provider had to assess, determine the necessity for, and refer to a specialist. Hospitals' reimbursement changed too. Medicare developed a payment methodology, a predetermined per case fee paid to the hospital. Managed care plans and some other third-party payors also began to negotiate other ways of paying hospitals. Competition was the word of the 1980s. For guaranteed volume, hospitals were negotiating per diem or per case fixed dollar income contracts with many managed care providers.

The effects of this change were great on hospitals. The philosophy of the managed care programs was to care for patients on an outpatient basis and limit the number of inpatient admissions and days. There was dramatic movement to the ambulatory care arena. This led to excess capacity of beds in all acute care facilities. An enormous decline in many hospitals' net income occurred.

The need to improve operating efficiencies became apparent. The new era demanded that hospitals become more aware of competition and that strategic planning and marketing were a necessity in their repertoire. That need transitioned into many different organizational structures, and product line management emerged.

REVIEW OF THE LITERATURE

Many executives of the hospital industry decided to review successful organization and management practices of other industries. Russ Coile, Jr., in his prediction of ten leading health care trends for the 1990s, described the success of product line management in other business and applied the concept to health care for the future. Mr. Coile focused on this model's ability to enhance production of a quality product in a cost-efficient manner. Accomplishing this goal will allow hospitals to contract with third-party payors for a total product, not component parts. Cole and Brown describe four product line management models in the health care industry.[2]

1. *Strategic business unit models* identify several business lines organized around clinical similarities.
2. *Distribution models* add to the responsibilities of existing line managers as product line managers.
3. *Market management models* create a sophisticated sales arm in the organization.
4. *Coordinated care models* create a new staff management position to increase the orientation to consumers.

Patterson and Thompson describe key organizational and operational attributes for three of these models.[3] The strategic business unit model decentralizes the management structure and gives total authority to the manager for the entire product. It has a product market orientation. This model provides an evaluation tool by measuring increases in profitability.

The distribution model provides an opportunity for line managers to assume additional responsibilities. It has a physician and market orientation with focus on channel placement. The evaluation tool is measuring an increase in utilization.

The market management model may not be as cost-effective since it layers on new staff management positions. It is market oriented in its identification of needs and opportunities. Its sophisticated sales arm focuses on volume. The evaluation of this model is through innovations in services and opportunities.

There have been numerous articles written about product line management. Most of them are inconclusive in their predictions of product line management becoming a dominant organizational structure in the health care arena. There seems to be some consistent themes in the literature that center around assessment, planning, change theory, human resources, transition, and evaluation.

Many authors encourage the health care executive to thoroughly assess their motives before changing to product line management. One of the areas all authors define as the most critical aspect of what must be done is appropriately defining the product line. Folger and Gee emphasize that true product lines have their focus on the marketplace.[4] A limitation of some of the nursing literature is that many of the articles are focused internal to the institution and describe nursing as a program line. This is in opposition to nursing being a component of services offered toward a total product.

Ernst and Whinney have made it very clear that functional departments are not product lines.[5] They outline nine criteria that establish an identifiable set of services that can be managed as a product line or a business. These are

1. Be identifiable to the market.
2. Have an identifiable market.
3. Contribute significantly to hospital long-range planning and daily operations.
4. Be an identifiable diagnostic category.
5. Have unique or dedicated production facilities, staff, and technology.
6. Be recognized as a unique or special program.
7. Be an administratively manageable unit.

8. Have linkage to treatment patterns of medical staff.
9. Parallel the organization of the medical staff.

Complete assessment of the present businesses and defining or reaffirming the mission are imperative steps to success. Once these steps are accomplished, a decision can be made about structure. This structure may be eclectic since most of the literature suggests that only a few services in the organization should be designed with a pure product line structure. A few authors oppose this and say that the entire hospital should go to product line in order to really achieve the goals of profitability and increased market share.

Most authors also identify three human resource issues as areas of caution. One is the choice of the product line manager. The characteristics and requirements of an effective product line manager are

- marketing understanding and savvy
- capability to champion a product
- entrepreneurial characteristics
- ability to assume decision-making power
- strategic planning, budgeting, and monitoring expertise

The second issue is gaining and maintaining the full support of the CEO in use of this concept. CEOs can get excited about product line management, but at a later time become complacent and perceived as unenthusiastic and unsupportive. It is imperative that the CEO live, eat, and breathe product line management if the change is to be successful.

The third area identified is the support rendered by staff involved in the product. Subtle innuendos and sabotage can occur. The product manager must be aware of this potential and make certain that early intervention occurs. All staff must be constantly reminded of their influence on the success of this change.

The literature varies in its approach to choice of PLM structure. One structure provides minimal disruption to the organization. It allows for the traditional organization to stay intact. Administrative function is maintained along functional department lines. There are then two options for the CEO as the institution moves to product line management. One is taking those same administrators and adding to their responsibilities one or more product lines for which they are accountable. Figure 6-1 illustrates this structure.

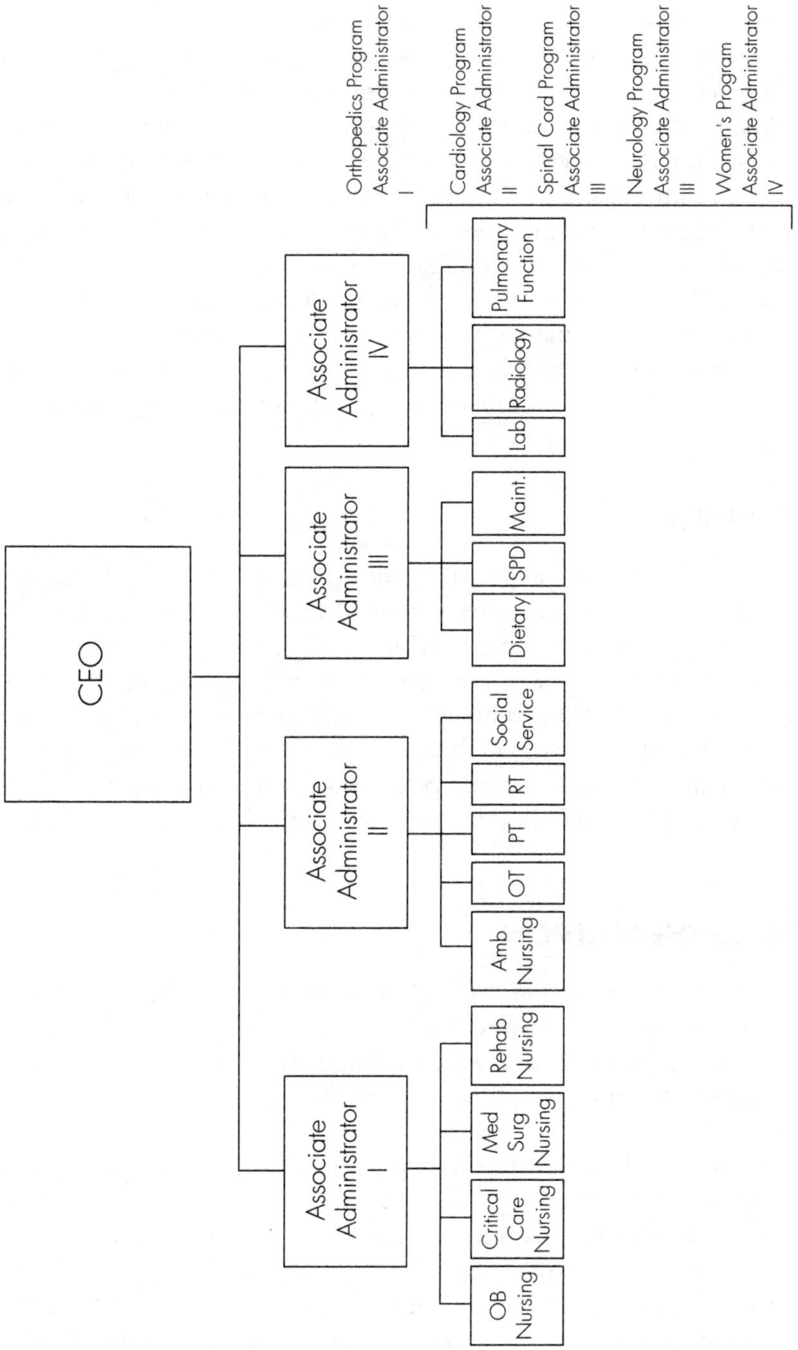

Figure 6-1 Functional Matrix

The second option (which layers administrative costs) is to use this same structure but hire new people to assume the PLM role. This structure becomes costly and may or may not pay for itself.

A third structure provides the opportunity for total reorganization. The traditional administrative structure is not maintained except for the support departments; that is, Plant Services, SPD, Dietary, etc. All clinical areas are totally decentralized and report to a product line manager. Figure 6-2 illustrates a totally reorganized structure.

A fourth structure gives all the extended continuum accountability to one product line manager. In this structure, all human resource support report to the product line manager for the product line but stay involved with their professional discipline. This focus is represented in Figure 6-3.

CASE STUDY

At Good Samaritan Regional Medical Center patients had received rehabilitation services and care for over 20 years. The Center enjoyed a reputation for exceptional care and innovation in the management of spinal cord and head injured patients. In the mid 1980s its market share began to be eroded. Many rehabilitation facilities were being developed in the Southwest and particularly in the county of this prestigious institute. It became apparent that competition was becoming strong and the once enjoyed position of primary provider of rehabilitation services was lost.

MAKING THE DECISION

In a strategic planning session, the hospital rehabilitation services were targeted as an area for review. Alternative solutions to the loss of market share and net income were explored. An in-depth assessment of the program through use of the product life cycle concept was completed.

The stages of the product life cycle include development, growth, shakeout, maturity, saturation, and decline. If a program has not been managed and is in the maturity, saturation, or decline stage, one must be concerned about petrification. If this has occurred, excess profit loss and market share loss are the outcomes. Then, divestiture, selling, bankruptcy, restructuring, or rebuilding are alternatives. As the rehabilitation

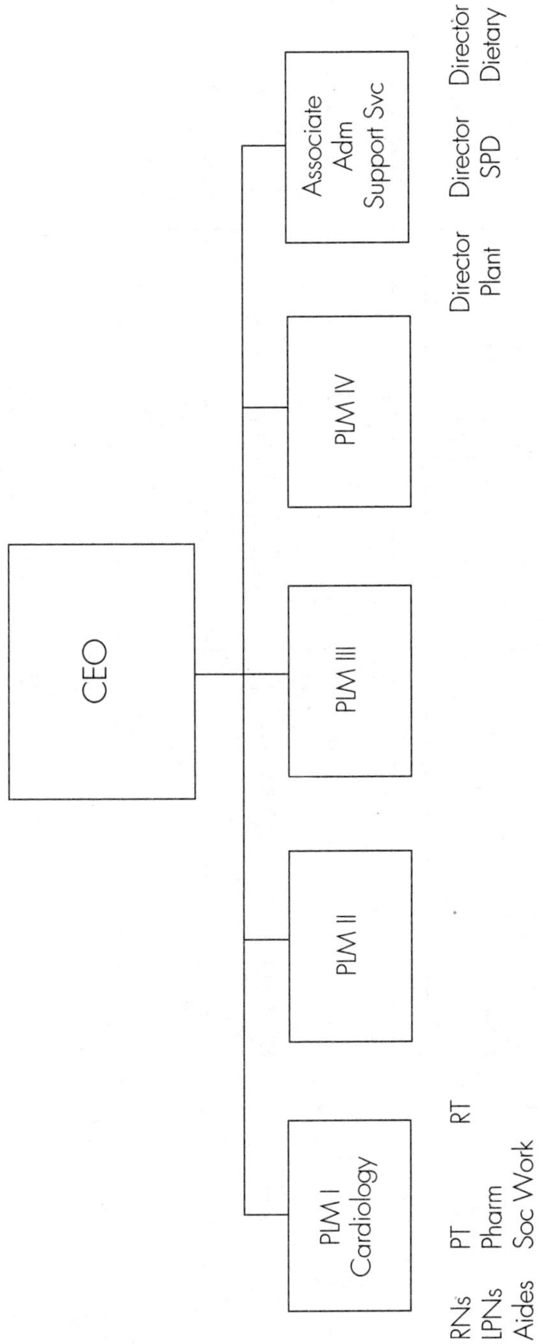

Figure 6-2 Pure Program Line Management

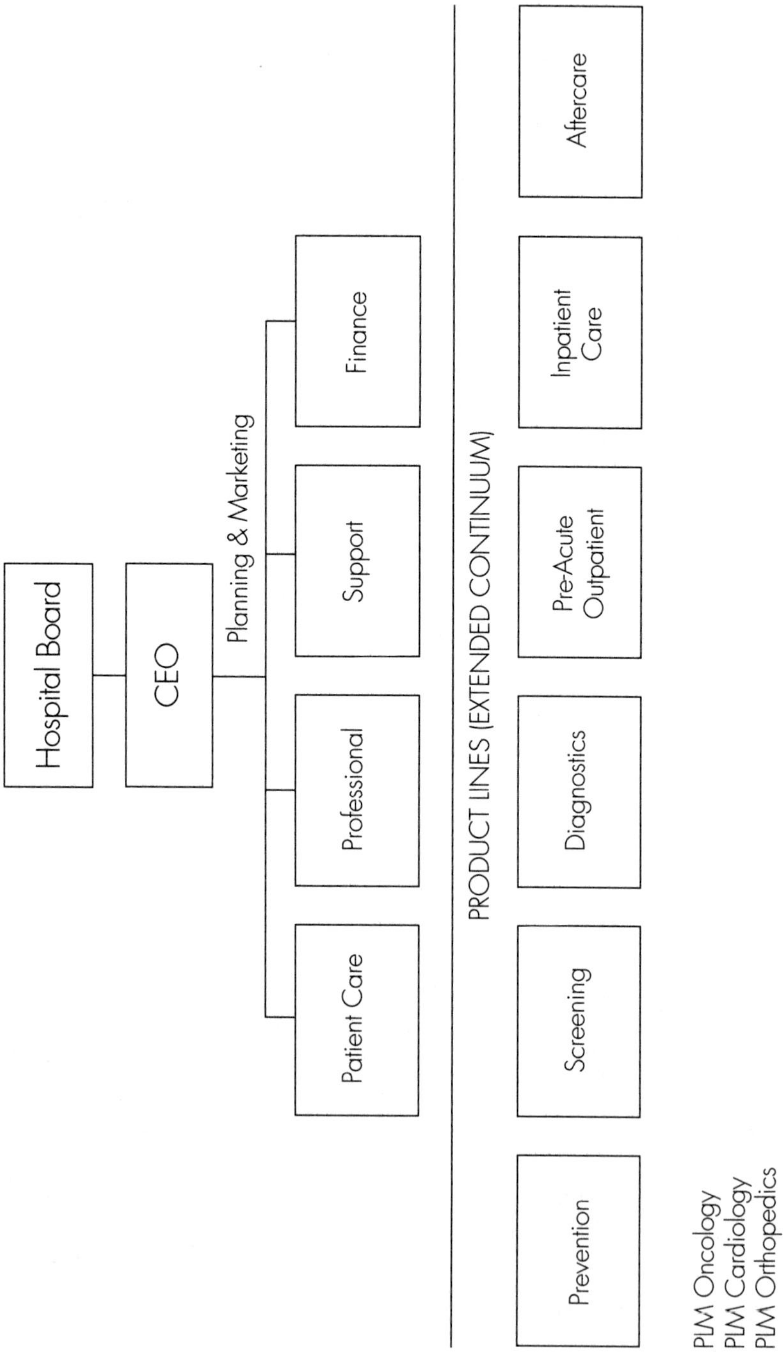

Figure 6-3 Product Lines (Extended)

program was analyzed, it was clear that decline had set in. Market share, profitability, and image were all measured in increasing negative percents over the past five years. The first question that was posed and answered was: How important is rehabilitation to the hospital mission? It was determined that as a tertiary center, with many spinal cord, orthopedic, and head injured patients generated from the Level I trauma status, rehabilitation was necessary to the mission. From that decision point until implementation, many activities occurred with little planning. It was decided (without a lot of discussion or input) that product line management was the organizational vehicle to making the rehabilitation services viable.

IMPLEMENTING THE NEW STRUCTURE

A massive restructure took place that eliminated all of the traditional department heads in physical therapy, speech therapy, nursing, recreational therapy, and occupational therapy. New positions and position descriptions were created on which all disciplines had the option to bid. These positions were called clinical coordinators and program supervisors. With this structure, 12 full-time middle managers were eliminated. A program line manager position for neuro and ortho/spinal cord was created. These were also available for bid. There seemed to be confusion by all involved on what was happening, why it was happening, and why so fast.

Within a period of two months, people were laid off, the new structure was waiting for implementation, and many professionals were wondering how they would function reporting to someone that was not of their same professional discipline. About six weeks into this process, the associate administrator held meetings with groups of rehabilitation staff on the goals of the change. These included improving marketability and resizing the human resources needed to manage these patients. It was also announced that over 50 full-time employees would be eliminated.

Staff were given no literature or detailed understanding of product line management. The next two weeks entailed many hours of interviews and selections for each of the new positions. During this time, continued attention to staff questions and concerns was primary. The staff continued to be confused about how this change would make a difference in their ability to attract or retain patients.

Implementation of the new structure took place two weeks later. All staff disciplines involved in the care of neurological patients reported through a program supervisor to a clinical coordinator. The theory was that they would all be very committed to the coordination and direct care of neuro-rehabilitation patients. It was also suggested that all services through home care would be provided, so that the extended product line concept would be incorporated. A marketing admissions director was hired to sell the total services of those three product lines and increase Samaritan's market share in those areas.

For one year, this concept and structure was continually refined and reorganized. The two program line manager positions were consolidated into one. Figure 6-4 illustrates this structure.

Months later coordinator and supervisor positions were consolidated and staff ended up divided into two groups—nurses and clinical support each reporting to a manager no matter what patient population they were treating. Staff uncertainty on structure and purpose issues remained predominant. Evaluation of success continued to focus on profitability and increase in market share. Neither of these areas had improved during this period.

ANALYSIS OF CASE

Since the institution had to make some dramatic changes to meet its financial and market share challenges, this move to product line management for rehabilitation services came about very fast. The depth of planning and coordinating within the organization was limited. The determination was to purely decentralize clinical services in the new model. An analysis of the four models described earlier in this chapter did not occur. The two basic philosophies used as alternatives were total decentralization or matrix.

The matrix approach does not disrupt employees or department heads as much as the decentralized model. It allows them to keep an identity with their professional peer group and helps them maintain a secure feeling. It also provides for better productivity, especially in an acute care setting. However, the matrix approach may not really give the message of focusing priorities in a different way. The "multiple boss" idea could provide confusion about who has what authority. It can also be confusing for the employees as they try to determine what they should do first, especially when more than one product line man-

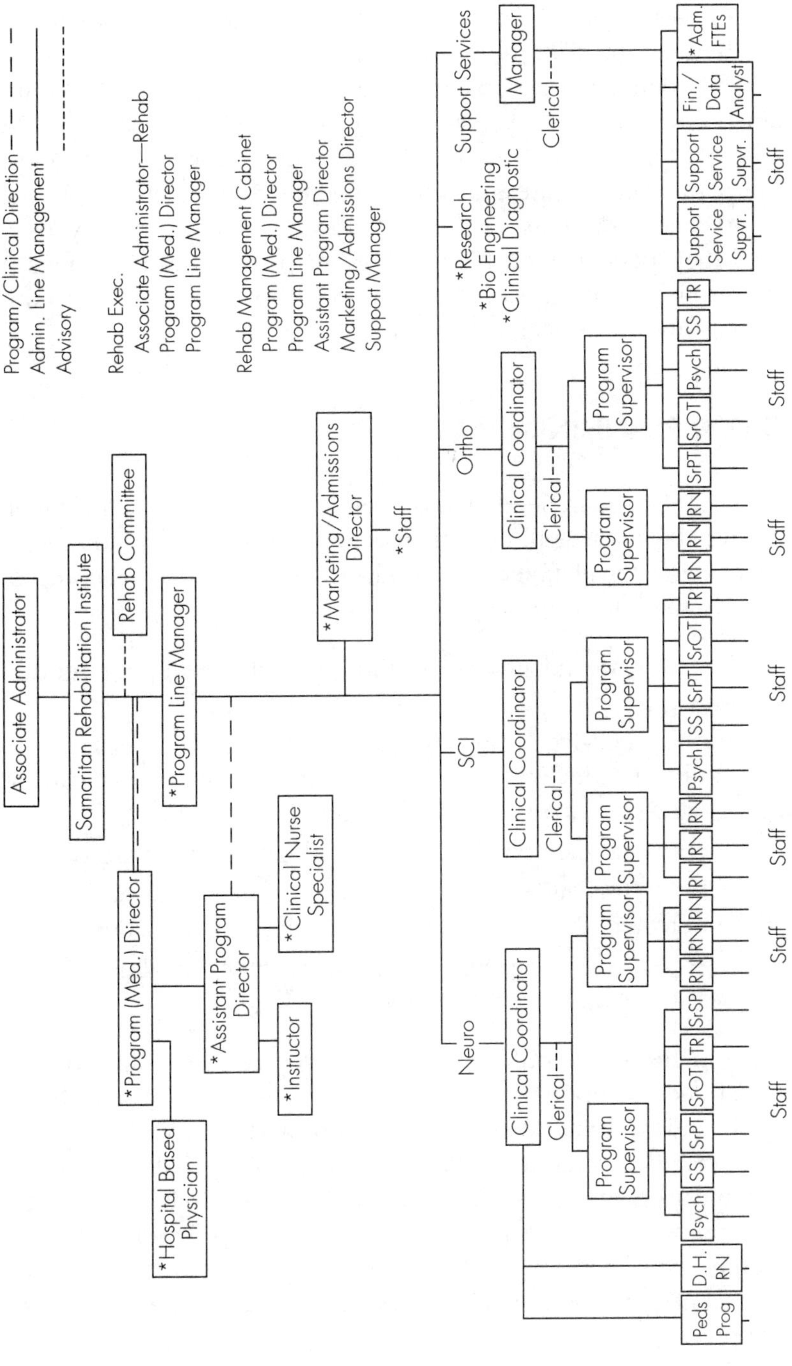

Figure 6-4 Rehabilitation Product Line

ager wants something accomplished. Department managers struggle with each other and with the product managers' priorities.

The decentralized approach works best in very specialized and contained areas; that is, psychiatric settings, rehabilitation settings. The message must be very clear to employees selected for these programs: they are to maximize care and profits for the patients of the product line. In the new structure, it is very difficult for these employees to establish their peer relationships with other professionals. Feelings of isolation from their profession are common. The decision to decentralize services in this case caused chaos.

NEED FOR PLANNING

An organized plan needed to be shared with the hospital managers and the rehabilitation staff. First, there should have been organizational decisions about the definition of product line. Product lines could be designed in the following ways:

1. diagnosis-related groups as the basis of developing product lines
2. strategic service groupings that take like diagnosis related groups and develop a product line from them; that is, cardiology-related, diagnosis-related groups
3. by managed care program; that is, all patients who are paid for by the same source
4. by outcome; that is, acute care, rehabilitation, outpatient
5. by extended line approach; that is, women's health including prenatal, acute hospital, posthospital care

Since there was not an organizational decision, rehabilitation services itself decided upon three product lines. Their lines were orthopedic rehabilitation, spinal cord rehabilitation, and neuro-rehabilitation. The lines included acute rehabilitation, day hospital rehabilitation, and some home care therapies. This provided the Rehabilitation Institute with marketing and contracting capabilities but begs the question of a continuum of care for orthopedic patients, spinal cord injury or neurologically damaged patients from prehospital through acute care and rehabilitation.

The confusion of other employees, physicians, and administrators within the whole organization was great. Questions arose about other rehabilitation services; that is, cardiology, pulmonary. Under what approaches are we functioning? Why product line management for three rehabilitation program lines? What are the functional efficiencies experienced by all departments of the acute care hospital? Should there be matrix management of three to four other strategic service groups; that is, oncology, cardiology, women's health, general surgery? The most important lesson learned in this case is to do a complete analysis of the entire institution and then develop a proposal for discussion and support by all administrators.

The proposed new structure should address its effect upon all areas of the institution in which product line management is being considered. Product line management is simply not the best approach for every hospital. It is predicted by some to be the future way of managing, but an informed, cautious approach to this decision is critical. It is considered by others to be "faddish" for health care institutions and not necessary to try.

SELECTING THE PRODUCT LINE MANAGER

The choice of a product line manager is crucial. A primary criteria for the manager is a clinical background such as nurse, social worker, or physician. Other criteria should be

- computer capability
- marketing skills
- managed care knowledge
- innovation
- financial knowledge and capability
- analytical skills
- if matrix format: must be able to work with multiple managers

If the manager does not have a clinical background, the focus of clinical outcomes will not be appropriately balanced with the marketing and sales aspects of the role. If there isn't balance and a clinical understanding of the patients' needs, the wrong decisions could be made about the product's production, restructuring, and the services that should be a part of the product.

PREPARING THE ORGANIZATION FOR CHANGE

How does an organization prepare for this change? First, management needs to understand and internalize change theory. This is a very difficult thing to accomplish, for it is a complex process that appears so simple. Management needs to remember there is an emotional and grieving process that accompanies any change. Because of this, a trouble-free environment will never occur. If the organization does not experience a level of discomfort, then the expected change has probably not occurred.

The stages encountered are

1. the present state, which is the ending of an era or ending a specific approach to something. The process experienced during this time is unfreezing.
2. the transition state, which is a time for completing the ending and developing increased energies for a new beginning. A period of "letting go" is experienced.
3. the desired state, where a new beginning occurs and the refreezing process is encountered by the organization.

THE RESPONSIBILITY OF MANAGERS

In changing to a product line structure, management needs to be responsible for the entire process. The first step includes explaining to the staff the history of the business being identified for this restructuring, what factors have positively or negatively affected the business, and why a new structure for managing the business is being planned. The staff will experience feelings of denial and may be immobilized. They may act overwhelmed and hope the new structure will disappear. The manager needs to direct this situation in order to avoid pure chaos.

The manager must share information about the expected change and repeat this information as often as possible. The visibility and rumor control role of the manager is imperative during this first stage of the process of change. The frustration that staff will experience cannot be minimized. Their anger, and the sense of knowing that things won't be the same, leads to negative attitudes about the organization, questions about personal need, satisfaction, and resistance. A real feeling of being out of control, along with inconsistent use of effective coping mechanisms, is to be expected.

This critical information sharing was entered into very late in the case study hospital. Four to six weeks after major decisions were made and announced, management had formal discussions with employees explaining the future. By that time, rumors and ideas of what was really going to happen had occurred and damage to morale and trust had begun. Staff knew that their volume was declining. They could have been helpful in shaping their future if they were brought into the process very early. Not enough time was allowed for staff involvement.

Managers can shape change into a positive experience by allowing staff participation in the design of their own future. This provides a new form of security. Staff must realize that "letting go" is key to their success. A manager helps this process by pointing out that old ways are no longer functional. This approach facilitates transition through stage two of the process of change.

The next stage provides opportunity for the staff to test some new behaviors. Analysis of what staff has been through and how it affects their future dispels the frustration and provides them with a high energy level. An important aspect of this phase is the flexibility of the manager. Flexibility is necessary in order to flow with some of the employee-generated new ideas. Managers must not cut off the energy, but refocus it toward the new structure and its goals as is necessary. By functioning in this fashion, the staff and the manager internalize the vision and incorporate a new reality into their behaviors.

Because of the limited staff meetings in the case study hospital, staff were bargaining with management and not really being creative in use of their ideas toward change. It took a few months after the first change for some of the supervisors, coordinators, and marketing employees to begin to contribute new thoughts and ideas to the proposal. Some of the changes occurred after the transition because of staff suggestions. However, other changes during the first year of product line management caused staff to continue their skepticism and hostility. There were so many changes without allowing for refreezing, that staff were continuously in the "letting go" phase. They would just let go of the previous security and begin to accept the new change when another change came about. They continued to be confused since "nothing seemed to work." In addition, their volume, image, and profitability continued to waiver. Staff were able to make it through the unfreezing stage but never accomplished refreezing.

ACQUIRING RESOURCES

In the implementation of product line management, some resources are needed that are different from those existing in the present organization. Before developing anything new, it is important to assess and answer the following questions:

1. How does the organization presently view the health care industry and how does this compare with the vision?
2. What are the roles and responsibilities of present managers and employees? How do those compare with the future roles and responsibilities?
3. What are the data resources available and how should they be formatted for the new business?
4. What is the present physical structure and how does it coordinate the flow of patients, employees, and information to support the new business?

In this case, the present organizational structure was reviewed. It was determined to be functional in nature, with traditional department heads. The new structure would develop various rehabilitation product lines. They were neurological, orthopedic, and spinal cord. Those lines each encompassed the acute rehabilitation phase through a home care program. A redesign of all services, including nursing, shifted the responsibility to one of those product lines and not to a functional department.

Roles and responsibilities were then examined. The functional role of a physical therapist, for example, was to provide physical therapy expertise to all patients. Under the new structure, therapists would work with a multidisciplinary team to provide the therapy *only* to orthopedic, neurologic, or spinal cord injured patients (depending on which product line manager had hired them).

DATA RESOURCES

As data resources were explored, the departmental accounting mechanism was found to be inadequate. The data needs were numerous. Display of information needed to be in a cost accounting methodology, based upon resources consumed by each individual product line. In order to make basic business decisions, it was also necessary to know managed care plan contract content and how the content applied to the reimbursement of each product line. Along with that information, the utilization by payor type of each product line was necessary. For example, information for the neurology product line included:

Payor	*% Cases*	*Payment Methodology*
Medicare	40%	Per Case
CIGNA	20%	Per Diem
AP/IPA	20%	% Charges
AHCCS	10%	Per Case
Self	5%	% Charges
Other	5%	Charges

Reports to review length of stay, market share, cost of services, and reimbursement are needed on a monthly basis. This information provides retrospective evaluation and allows for projecting the future, altering expenses, and determining if the marketing plan is being appropriately implemented or needs alteration.

ORGANIZATION AND PHYSICIAN DESIGN NEEDS

A review of the flow of patients is also necessary. This entails examining how patients access the facility and engage in the services provided. What are the barriers to a smooth, easy flow of the patient through the system? What written documentation should accompany the patient? The new system should be easily accessible, with the patient registered once and then identified each consecutive time service is requested. The patient encounters, by any team member, should be recorded so the cost accounting documents accurately reflect the time and cost of the encounter. Patients, families, physician, and staff should be aware of what outcomes the services are expected to produce. The outcomes then need measurement to assure clinical and cost-effective care.

PREPARING FOR NEW ROLES

The next steps involve preparing position descriptions and hiring into the new positions. It is very important to do this step as formally as possible. Position descriptions need to be written to accurately reflect the new roles and responsibilities. Qualifications must be made very clear when hiring, and must be emphasized and maintained. If this does not happen, staff will be further confused as they encounter the stages of the change process. In order for staff to understand this reality, formal interviews of all internal and external candidates must occur. Appointments to this position are made from the group of applicants. Present staff cannot just be rearranged and given new positions. If this is done, the organization may experience more than normal resistance to this new concept of managing the business. Once appointments to new positions are made, a date for implementation can be identified. All preparation of staff, physicians, and patients should be completed prior to implementation. As part of implementation, a formal orientation to the new position must occur. Checkpoints on a weekly basis assure management that previously established goals are being met and allow for adjustments when necessary. Weekly meetings with employees provide a vehicle for ventilation of concerns, modifying the process, and strengthening interdisciplinary working relationships.

IMPACT UPON NURSING

How does all this affect nursing? A major risk could be a decrease in the role nursing really should have in identifying and insuring standards of nursing and quality of care. Generally the nurse, more than any other discipline, has a total picture of the patients, their needs, and expected outcome of their illness. If nursing's role is defined to maintain the vision for the product and continue to shape the cost and quality of the product, the product line management approach can be successful. However, if nursing's role is superseded by a manager who is so heavily focused on marketing the product, then the model will fail.

Nurses need to be recognized for their multitalented abilities. They can be good business persons who link cost and quality in a very positive way. Nurses can best visualize the product being developed, implemented, and evaluated. They can describe the expected product and the services of which that product is a part. If the philosophy and structure support those statements, nursing will continue to thrive under product line management. If the philosophy and structure support more of a "piecework" approach to product development, nursing's role could be virtually eliminated.

The 1991 Joint Commission standards may provide a safety net to correct this potential loss of nursing process and standards. JCAHO NC Standard 3 criteria states that the nurse executive and other appropriate registered nurses develop hospital-wide patient care programs, policies, and procedures that describe how the nursing care needs of patients or patient populations are assessed, evaluated, and met. The nurse executive is required to be accountable for nursing standards, care, and quality throughout the organization in spite of direct line authority. In a total or partial product line structure, this requires very concentrated organized coordination of activities between and among the nursing department and product line assigned nurses.

It would be advisable for the nurse executive to negotiate the following with other administrators:

- time commitments from PLM who need to be educated to nursing's goals and standards
- time commitments from the nursing staff in PLM assignments for committee work in developing standards, policy and procedure, education competencies, and QA indicators and monitoring
- written reports from the nurses in PLM on a quarterly basis about their completion of goals and expectations in relationship to the standards
- quarterly QA reports through the nursing QA structure for formal action and nursing practice oversight

This decade is exciting and challenging. Due to the many changes in health care, nurses and nursing need to be flexible and visionary. Product line management may or may not be here permanently. No matter what the new structure, professional nursing must provide the core standards for each clinical product. Nursing must continue to gain credibility in its business acumen and must help the health care industry shape the future.

NOTES

1. Andersen, Arthur & Company and the American College of Hospital Administrators. (1984). *Health Care in the 1990's: Trends and Strategies.* Chicago: Arthur Andersen & Company and ACHA.
2. Cole, G. and Brown, C. (1988). Product line management: Concept to reality. *Topics in Health Care Financing,* 14(3), 62–75.

3. Ernst and Whinney. (1983). *Strategic Program Unit Planning: Strategies and Management Tools for a Product-Oriented Market Place*. Chicago: Ernst & Whinney.
4. Folger, J.C. and Gee, E.P. (1987). *Product Management for Hospitals: Organizing for Profitability*. Chicago: American Hospital Publishing.
5. Patterson, D.J. and Thompson, K.A. (1987). Product line management: Organization makes the difference. *Healthcare Financial Management*, February, 66–72.

BIBLIOGRAPHY

Anderson, R.A. (1985). Products and product line management in nursing. *Nursing Administration Quarterly*, 10(1), 65–67.

Bird, G.A. (1988). Product line management and nursing. *Nursing Management*, 19(5), 46–48.

Cassak, D. (1986). Extended product line-preparing for the consumer revolution in healthcare. *Health Industry Today*, June, 12–16.

Charns, M.P. and Smith, L.J. (1989). Product line management and continuum of care. *Health Matrix*, 7(1), 40–49.

Droste, T. (1988). Product line management: Misunderstood, feared. *Hospitals*, July 5, 30–31.

Foittier, M.D. and Repasky, L.J. (1988). Attitudes of hospital executives toward product line management: A pilot survey. *Health Care Management Review*, 13(3), 15–22.

Goodrich, R.G. (1985). St. Luke's Hospital reaps benefits by using product line management. *Modern Healthcare*, February 15, 157–158.

Johnson, J.E., Arvidson, A.C., Costa, L.L., Hekhuis, F.M., Lennox, L.A., Marshall, S.B., and Moran, M.J. (1987). Marketing your nursing product line; reaping the rewards. *JONA*, 17(11), 29–33.

Johnson, R.R. and McGinty, D.B. (1989). Product line management requires change in financial reports. *Healthcare Financial Management*, August, 43(8), 34–42.

Kanter, R.M. (1983). *The Change Masters*. New York: Simon and Schuster.

Lowe, L. (1987). How to avoid chaos in the transition to product line management. *Health Care Strategic Management*. April, 5(4), 9–13.

Nachel, J.G., Fenarolli, P.J., and Kis, G. (1987). Product line performance reporting: A key to cost management. *Healthcare Financial Management*, November, 41(11), 54–62.

Nachel, J.G. and Kues, I.W. (1986). Product line management: Systems and strategies. *Hospital and Healthcare Services Administration, March/April*, 109–123.

Patterson, D. and Porn, L. *Program/Product Line Evaluation*. American College of Healthcare Executives.

Perlman, D. and Takacs, G.J. (1990). The ten stages of change. *Nursing Management*, 21, 33–38.

Peters, T. and Austin, N. (1985). *A Passion for Excellence*. New York: Random House.

Salter, V. (1986). Product line management: Its meaning and future promise. *Health Care Strategic Management,* May, 13–15.

Sloate, S. *Product Line Management.* Shands Hospital, Gainesville, FL.

VanDoren, D.C. and Spielman, A.P. (1989). Hospital marketing: Strategy reassessment in a declining market. *Journal of Health Care Marketing,* 9(1), 15–24.

Ward, M.J. and Moran, S.G. (1984). Resistance to change: Recognize, respond, overcome. *Nursing Management,* 15, 30–33.

Weber, J.R. (1986). Product lines in hospitals. *HC&C,* January, 36–39.

Yano-Fong, D. (1988). Advantages and disadvantages of product line management. *Nursing Management,* May, 27–31.

CHAPTER 7

From the Vision to the Reality: Developing a Shared Governance Structure

Porter-O'Grady and Finnegan's (1984)[1] watershed book described a new organizational structure for nursing organizations. Its advent signaled the beginning of a proliferation of a significant body of nursing and hospital literature concerning the role of the professional nurse in the decision making of health care organizations. Over 1,050 hospitals across the country have either expressed an interest in the implementation of this new organizational structure, or are in the process of implementation. In addition, studies such as the Magnet Hospital Study of the American Academy of Nursing,[2] the Institute of Medicine Study,[3] and the work of the National Commission on Nursing Implementation Project[4] all point to the need to recruit and retain nurses by restructuring the nursing workplace to reflect greater nurse participation. The proliferation of literature and the extent of the activity surrounding shared governance suggests that it is indeed a significant step in the evolution of professional nursing and is a movement that is here to stay.

This chapter describes the implementation of a shared governance model in the acute care hospital. It is a composite of the experiences of several organizations. A brief theoretical overview of the concepts central to shared governance is presented first. The implementation of a councilor model is described, including discussions of pertinent project management issues. The realities of a major organizational change are emphasized, with descriptions of both successful strategies and implementation errors.

THEORETICAL FOUNDATIONS

Participation

Greater staff nurse involvement in patient care decisions is strongly advocated as one strategy to increase retention and satisfaction while improving the quality of patient care. It is believed that increased nurse participation in decisions that affect patient care will meet certain needs. These include the demands of nurses for greater control over nursing practice and their expectations for professional partnerships in the delivery of patient care.

Professional nurses possess not only nursing knowledge but also information about the reality of providing care within the organizational environment. Participative structures allow the health care organization to benefit from the knowledge of these professionals in the identification and the resolution of patient care problems. The involvement of professional nurses in patient care decisions will strengthen both the quality of care and the financial well-being of the organization.

Participation is broadly defined in the organizational and nursing literature. One of the more useful definitions identifies the arena in which participation may occur and also the people involved. Nurse participation in health care organizations can fall into four broad and overlapping areas:

1. goal setting
2. decision making
3. problem solving
4. participating in the change process[5,6]

Participation may be centered in the individual, a nurse-manager pair, a group of nurses, or a multidisciplinary team. The group may or may not have manager representation.

The manner in which participation is operationalized in health care organizations varies considerably. However, all of the strategies applied reflect a common philosophy. The focus of control for certain decisions is shifted downward to those individuals actually doing the work of patient care.

Quality circles are one example of a participative structure that is enjoying some attention in the nursing literature. Small groups of nurses meet together regularly to solve problems that affect the day-to-day delivery of care on a nursing unit. Solutions are then recommended to management for implementation.[7]

Joint goal setting is another example of strategy to enhance participation in the workplace. For example, organizations that use the "management by objectives" approach give professional nurses the opportunity to define the focus of their patient care performance.[8]

Nurse-physician committees can also be considered to be participative structures, if the staff nurse is a valid member of such groups. This is not always the case.

Finally, shared governance decision-making structures are implemented, which define participation through the vested authority of the professional nursing staff for certain clinical decisions. This is clearly the strongest level of participation and the most complicated to administer. Differences in participation methods, by location and degree of participation, are summarized in Table 7-1.

Table 7-1 Forms of Professional Nurses Participation in Contemporary Nursing Organizations

Level of Participation	*Method of Participation*	*Degree of Participation*
Individual	Management by objectives	Low
	Delivery system role	High
	Nurse peer review program	Medium
	Shared council membership governance	High
Work Group	Quality circles	Low
	Unit-based quality assurance	Medium
	Manager/staff project teams	Medium
	MD/RN joint committees	Medium
Organizational	Councilor model of shared governance	High
	Unification model of shared governance	High
	Unit-based model of shared governance	High

It is critical for nursing leaders to carefully consider the location and degree of participation to be achieved by introducing participative structures. Failure to define the boundaries of nurse participation in the beginning can result in significant authority conflicts between administration and staff, and heightened dissatisfaction. This is a common error in project conception and selection.

There are many ways to increase nurse participation. Shared governance structures are the most comprehensive and complete. If implementation is to be successful, shared governance structures must be distinguished from the lesser authority and accountability of participative management structures and processes. Shared governance is *not* the same as participative management. It is a decision-making structure that vests real authority in the decision making of the professional nurse.

There is a discrepancy in the hospital administrative literature and the nursing literature regarding the degree of participation needed in the professional nursing workplace. Nursing leaders can be caught between demands of the nursing staff for greater participation, and the beliefs of health care administrators who value the maintenance of the status quo.[9] This may be further complicated by the fact that the professional staff is unclear about what decisions they want to participate in, or how much time they want to spend in decision-making activities.

The goal in designing an effective shared governance structure is to select and design a structure that meets the demands of both groups.[10] The construction of a shared governance system must assure the administrator, through documented outcomes, that the shared governance structure not only enhanced patient care but made it more cost-effective. At the same time, staff nurses must be able to see the tangible evidence of shared governance decisions upon their nursing practice.

Organizational research has consistently documented the benefits of employee participation on worker performance and productivity. Miller and Monge (1986) found, in a meta-analysis of 106 studies, a positive correlation between participation and productivity improvements.[11] However, the actual relationship between productivity and participation is not well understood. Some argue that productivity is enhanced through participation because diverse groups are forced to coordinate their efforts through increased teamwork.[12] Others argue that goal setting in participative structures results in intense commitment to more difficult goals, which produces increased productivity in the long run.[13]

Participation is defined differently by various researchers. Also, the effects of participation upon performance are blurred by the influence of other factors. For example, Wagner and Gooding (1987), in another meta-analysis, found that participative structures were often accompanied by other workplace satisfiers, such as pay and benefit improvements. In addition, the implementation of a participative structure produces a by-product of increased manager attention to employees, which itself has a strong influence on productivity.[14]

When identifying the needs to be addressed through the implementation of shared governance, productivity outcomes should be identified by the project team. These are then included in the design of project evaluation methods. Productivity goals are included in those approaches used to acquire administrative support for the restructuring project.

AUTHORITY

Shared governance means shared professional authority. Unfortunately, many nursing organizations suffer from a lack of authority structures which allow for the full application of nursing expertise to patient care decisions. For professionals, authority is derived from a body of scientific knowledge. Within nursing organizations, the actual delivery of nursing care is determined by the knowledge, skill, and judgment of the professional nurse. Therefore, the organization's authority structure must provide the professional nurse with a certain accountability for patient care decisions.

Authority issues within the shared governance structure are commonly defined through a rational democratic model. All members of the nursing organization are seen as politically equal with equal authority, under the principles of competence, representativeness, and efficiency. However, individual authority may be limited by competency.[15] Some nurses, by virtue of their expertise, will be given more authority over certain patient care decisions.

The professional nursing staff should be the source of nursing practice standards within the organization, just as the American Nurses Association is the external source of nursing standards. In shared governance structures, the authority of individual nurses is shared with democratically elected representatives of the professional nursing staff. Peer review represents the authority of professional nursing groups within an organization, to reward or punish professional nurses' performance.[16]

Clearly, the shift in authority under shared governance is a crucial change experience. Traditionally, the nursing management team maintained authority for both clinical and operational decision making. Since nursing organizations have tended to promote their best clinicians into management positions, the incorporation of clinical decision making into management roles is not surprising.

If authority for clinical decision making is truly transferred to the professional nursing staff, then managers will be left with a much stronger operational authority. Theoretically, this change would result in increased manager accountability for operations. The management team performance would improve. However, if these individuals have significant deficits in management knowledge and expertise, management performance will not excel. In fact, there may be strong manager opposition to the implementation of shared governance, because of the potential loss of the only area of responsibility in which some managers feel truly competent: clinical decision making.

In shared governance organizations, new authority is vested in the professional work of nurses. Each individual nurse must recognize and accept authority for the implementation of the professional nursing role. Since there are differences in educational preparation and experience level, the exercise of professional nursing authority requires differentiated roles.[17]

SHARED GOVERNANCE

Both the nursing and organizational behavior literature contain many references to certain key concepts, which combine to form the conceptual framework for shared governance structures. These can be grouped into beliefs about people, leadership expectations, and workplace values.

Beliefs About People

Porter-O'Grady and Finnegan (1984), in their landmark work on shared governance, described the essential conflict experienced by professional nurses who are the employees of modern health care organizations. The hierarchical structure of most nursing organizations provides obstacles to the application of professional judgment. Indeed, professional judgment must sometimes supersede organizational policy, in the interests of quality patient care.[18]

Many professional nurses experience a lack of control over their nursing work, a sense of meaninglessness about their profession, and an isolation from their colleagues. This is due to organizational structures that do not provide the information necessary to make good decisions. There is a paucity of reward systems that recognize both needs for professional achievement and economic security.[19] Also, many health care organizations are designed with little appreciation for nursing's contribution to patient care. The environment of such organizations includes a simmering distrust about the capacity of nurses to make good decisions.

Shared governance structures operate from the belief that nurses are good and worthy of trust. If given the opportunity *and* the resources, professional nurses are able to make good decisions. These structures are designed so that the professional nursing staff sees itself as unified over a common goal, individuals are valued, communication is pervasive, and decision making is open and participative. The nursing organization shifts from "command to consensus."[20]

For example, Peters and Austin, in their 1985 follow-up work on leadership and excellence, extensively discussed the philosophies of organizations that valued their people.[21] All of the organizational philosophies contained certain core beliefs that have application to nursing shared governance:

1. Nurses do not dislike work. Participate with them in defining nursing work and they will achieve excellence in patient care. Nurses expect partnerships.
2. Nurses are more likely to seek opportunities to increase their competency when the demands for improvement come from their peers rather than from management. This exemplifies professional self-governance.
3. Nurses are individuals with unique ego and individual needs. To the extent that these are satisfied in the professional workplace, they will be committed to it.

4. Nurses cannot be motivated by anyone else. The workplace can only provide the stimulation for self-respect, self-confidence, and ongoing self-assessment.
5. Nurses expect rewards to be tied to performance.
6. When nurses perceive themselves to be in an atmosphere of trust, they will put themselves at risk through challenging the status quo and developing creative solutions to patient care problems.

Peters and Austin (1985) provide a good example of participating with workers in the definition of their work.[22] In a Ford Motor Company, every assembly line worker was given a button that could shut down the line. The worker could do this if necessary to make an adjustment. Many fears were expressed about the negative consequences of this change upon overall productivity. Buttons were indeed pushed, some twenty to thirty times a day! However, the shutdown lasted only ten seconds. Quality adjustments were made during those ten seconds.

The overall productivity of the assembly line was found to have neither increased nor decreased. However, there were dramatic increases in quality. The number of defects per car was reduced from 17.1 to .8. The number of cars requiring rework after coming off the line dropped by 97% and the number of union grievances plummeted from well over 200 to an average of less than 12 a month![23] By giving workers control over some of their work, quality improvements were achieved.

The power of giving professional nurses control over their practice cannot be overlooked in today's health care environment. Increasingly, health care organizations are being scrutinized and graded on their ability to provide quality patient care. An enormous quality and utilization review industry has developed in response to consumer and payor demands for cost-effective care. The economic viability of health care organizations rests upon passing this scrutiny. What nursing organization would not be happy with the achievement of improvements in quality similar to those described in the Ford Motor Company example?

Shared governance structures are producing these achievements. Instead of buttons, nursing organizations are being restructured so that no decision about patient care is even considered without the equal participation of the professional nursing staff.

The basic people beliefs embodied in a shared governance structure are illustrated in Exhibit 7-1. The acceptance of these beliefs re-

Exhibit 7-1 People Beliefs in Shared Governance Structures

- Nurses are good and worthy of trust.
- Professional nurses are self-governing.
- Individual needs must be recognized and valued.
- Professional nurses expect partnerships and participation.
- Professional nursing judgment is essential to the provision of quality care.

quires that nurses are no longer seen as employees but as self-governing professionals.

Leadership Beliefs

The expectations of leaders in a shared governance environment parallel those characteristics attributed to transformational leaders.[24] These characteristics were discussed in greater detail earlier. The top nursing leader must be charismatic and motivating because the development and maintenance of a shared governance structure demands a strong personal and professional investment from all of the professional nursing staff.

The nursing leadership group, in a shared governance organization, is committed to the primary goal of assuring the support of nursing practice. Because commitment to nursing governance must pervade all levels of the organization, leadership emerges in every distinct area where nursing services are provided.

Finally, leaders in a shared governance organization are seen as teachers. These individuals not only identify opportunities to apply concepts of advanced nursing practice, but allow for organizational learning.

The shift of clinical decisions to the practicing nurse requires that participants understand the behavior of health care organizations. Mistakes will be made, because the bedside nurse is rarely exposed to this reality. When errors do occur, nursing leaders must see the mistakes as opportunities for greater education about the health care organization.

If these leadership attributes are present, continual transformation to greater levels of excellence in practice are sure to follow. Those nursing leaders whose educational preparation contains both advanced nursing practice and organizational theory will be prepared to successfully meet these new leadership expectations. The expectations of leaders in a shared governance organization are outlined in Exhibit 7-2.

Work Place Values

The emergence of shared governance organizations is one of nursing's responses to the demands of the contemporary health care environment. With the implementation of effective governance structures, the health care organization is able to maximize access to its most valuable asset: the professional knowledge and judgment of professional nurses.

The predominant values in the professional work place of a shared governance organization are easily identified. The work place is structured in a manner that values the strong definition and differentiation of nursing roles.[25] The boundaries and accountabilities of nursing are defined and operationalized through the continual redefinition of nursing job descriptions, career ladders, and performance systems. The process of continual redefinition reflects a recognition that the practice of nursing is a dynamic and evolving art and science.

Unfortunately, many contemporary nurses practice in professional work places that differ dramatically from the one previously described. Financial pressures have resulted in many health care organizations cutting back on support services, such as housekeeping and transportation. Similarly, ancillary patient care services, such as the lab and respiratory therapy, are being equally down-sized in response to economic demands. The result is chaos, due to imbalanced and understaffed patient

---

Exhibit 7-2 Expectations of Leaders in a Shared Governance Organization

- Charismatic and Motivating
- Teachers
- Facilitators of Nursing Practice
- Leaders in all arena of practice
- Transformational

care systems. Most of the workload from these down-sized departments becomes informally integrated into the nursing role. Problems in the delivery of patient care increase and must be repeatedly addressed every day. In this case, not only is nursing accountability blurred, but nurses are often the ones who take the responsibility for patching the system together in order to meet patient needs.[26]

In a shared governance organization, nursing does not take on the accountability of other patient care departments. This does not mean that there is not pressure to take on the work. However, the top nursing leader is more likely to withstand these demands because of the presence of clearly defined nursing roles and identified cost-effective outcomes.

Another value in the shared governance work place is reflected in the importance placed upon professionally defined relationships over hierarchically defined ones. Nurses engage in purposeful and equally collaborative relationships with all groups for the benefit of patient care. For example, joint physician-nurse committees collaborate to solve patient care problems. Practicing nurses and managers engage in partnerships through new participative decision-making structures. The nurse-patient relationship is no longer determined by sets of policy and procedures but by professional standards. Problem solving is based upon the assumption that complex issues need to be resolved at the local level: the bedside.[27] There is less of a distinction between administrative and practice accountabilities. Delivery systems are designed to emphasize the collaborative nature of professional relationships. The patient medical record is integrated in a truly collaborative and professional environment.

The collaborative nature of the professional work place in a shared governance organization results in a networking environment. People are talking to one another. Nursing groups are no longer isolated from one another. People, information, and other resources are freely shared. The communication system is structured for speed and efficiency because of the value placed on strategic information sharing. Networks will emphasize equal participation, lateral communication, multidisciplines, and informality.[28] Everyone wins, including the patient.

The empowerment of the individual professional will ultimately produce the attainment of superior quality care. The predominant values of the shared governance work place are illustrated in Exhibit 7-3.

Exhibit 7-3 Predominant Values in a Shared Governance Workplace

- A priority for well-defined nursing roles and accountabilities
- Pre-eminence of professionally defined relationships between nurses and others
- Respect for the collaboration of professional groups
- Value for the multidisciplinary nature of patient care
- Support for decision making at the point of service
- A priority for efficient communication
- The importance of equal participation
- Respect for strategic information sharing
- A value for all disciplines

The Councilor Model

One of the earliest shared governance structures was developed by O'Grady and Finnegan (1984) and successfully implemented at St. Joseph's Hospital in Atlanta, Georgia. This structure calls for the development of participative "councils" which are believed to encompass all of the key decision-making activities within a nursing organization. These councils include: a Nursing Management Council, a Nursing Education Council, a Nursing Quality Assurance Council, a Nursing Practice Council, and a Nursing Executive Council. Staff nurses act as members and chairpersons of all but the Nursing Management Council.[29]

Nursing bylaws are developed, which delineate how the councils function under the structure and legitimize the governance model within the health care organization. Bylaws identify to the board of directors that which nursing is held accountable for in the delivery of care. Each element of the nursing organization is defined, along with its authority, accountability, system maintenance, and support. The degree and kind of participation is clearly identified. Well-defined nursing bylaws aid in the organization and coordination of the shared governance system.[30]

Bylaws also pave the way for nursing representation on the board of directors. The appointment of a nurse to the board of directors gives the nursing organization influence over the overall direction of the organization, defining its mission and evaluating the cost-effective outcomes of the organization.[31] This relationship recognizes the equal partnership of nurses in the delivery of care and values the perspective and insights that nurses bring to patient care problem solving.

PROJECT MANAGEMENT ISSUES

Project Conception

It is assumed that nursing leaders who contemplate the implementation of a shared governance model are interested in the growth and development of a professional nursing practice environment. Consequently, project conception begins with the identification of problems believed to be obstacles to the attainment of this goal.

Most organizations begin with a restructuring project team, which has the responsibility to identify present problems and their potential solutions. Clinical and management leaders must be part of this team, along with staff nurses. The staff nurse participants will provide the real-world feedback about the limitations of certain solutions. The top nursing administrator should chair the group.

The decision-making structure of a nursing organization is one central piece of a professional practice environment. Since shared governance is an alternative decision-making structure, the project team must ask certain questions about the performance of the present organizational structure. How are decisions being made? Evaluation may reveal that present nursing committees are poorly attended and ineffective. The nursing organization may be spending lots of time fixing decisions made in haste by an overloaded management team. Creative and pro-active decision making may be limited by the present structure because of layers of hierarchy and cumbersome policies. The daily organization of nursing work may be inadequate to meet current demands.

This assessment is then converted into goals for a new nursing structure:

- to balance autonomy and direction
- to refine current information flow
- to create more opportunities for nurse participation
- to improve the quality of nursing department decisions
- to increase the productivity of the nursing department
- to improve the quality of care

In addition, the nursing leader may evaluate the organizational structure for its effect upon the delivery of professional nursing services. A delivery system that allows the organization to effectively utilize nursing knowledge and expertise is a second component of a professional practice environment. Do nurses see the organization as one which has an environment supporting professional practice? What is the reputation of the nursing department in the community? How many vacant positions are there? Are nurses involved in the organization? Is the delivery system designed to effectively match nursing expertise with patient characteristics? The answers to these questions could produce additional goals for a new nursing structure:

- to promote organizational commitment
- to clarify the purpose for nursing work
- to define nursing within the larger organization
- to re-align nursing roles to reflect nursing work
- to encourage individual and professional growth

The next level of assessment concerns the organization's readiness for change and the environment's ability to support a new direction for nursing. An organization culture that promotes excellence and innovation is the third element of a professional practice environment. Since transformation to a shared governance structure occurs over a three- to five-year period, this evaluation is central to project success. Is the organization comfortable with change? How is participation viewed, in general, by the organizational leadership? If other department heads do not value staff participation, this viewpoint may produce opposition to nursing's new direction. Who has the power to move the change through the organization? Who can block progress? Who holds the financial purse strings?

Do the identified goals fit with the overall mission of the organization? It may be that the mission and the philosophy of the hospital will fit better with a certain type of shared governance structure. How is the nursing organization viewed by the rest of the organization? How would a participative nursing structure fit with this perception?

What are the performance expectations for the nursing department? Would changing to a shared governance structure aid in the achievement of these expectations? If the nursing department is not seen as performing well, other needs may take precedence over the implementation of shared governance.

At the end of the project conception phase the project team will have identified problems and their potential solutions in relation to the nursing organization's decision-making structure, delivery system, and organizational culture.

Project Selection

What should be the focus of the restructuring project? This question is the central issue of the project selection team. The decision-making structure, the delivery system, and the organizational environment are all examined as potential targets. Should one, two, or all three areas be targeted for change? Which shall be first?

If a shared governance decision-making structure is selected, then significant resources will be required. Is there a stable administrative team that will be able to see the project to completion? The stability of the hospital administration team is crucial to the maintenance of support for the new structure. Are the financial resources of the hospital able to support the education and the staff participation required for structure development and maintenance? What is the educational and skill mix of the present nursing staff? Is there a sufficient knowledge base in the theory and practice of professional nursing?

Similarly, does the organization show its support for the advancement of nursing practice through the presence of clinical nurse specialists? The advanced nursing practice preparation of these individuals provides a valuable and crucial resource to the implementation of shared governance. Clinical nurse specialists not only support the facilitation of change, but also can provide significant help in the delineation and definition of nursing practice within the organization.

A shared governance structure cannot be implemented without the skills of an effective management team. The complexity of an alteration in the organization structure requires that these individuals are strong practitioners of nursing administration. This strength is evidenced by the presence of up-to-date and efficient operational systems and the educational preparation of the nursing management team.

After an extensive organizational assessment, a decision is made to restructure one of the three components of a professional nursing practice environment. A shared governance structure will be selected under certain conditions. There must be strong administrative and organizational support for the transfer of real clinical decision-making authority to professional nurses. There must be dedicated resources to the project. The organization must possess or be able to obtain the requisite nursing knowledge necessary for the implementation of shared governance. The management team must be effective. Finally, the shared governance structure must fit with the organizational environment.

Planning

The project team is given the responsibility for developing the implementation and evaluation plan for the change. Activities are directed towards the implementation of the five major governance councils. The Nursing Practice Council is vested with the authority to make clinical nursing practice decisions. The Nursing Management Council assures that operational systems support nursing practice and will facilitate the decisions of the other councils. The Nursing Education Council assures that educational activities meet the needs of the nursing staff. The Nursing Quality Assurance Council vests professional nurses with the authority over all activities that affect the quality of patient care. The Executive or Governance Council coordinates the efforts of the other four councils and provides strategic direction.[32] The decision making is shared in each council by a representative membership of each area of the nursing organization, managers, and advanced nursing practitioners.

Several difficult decisions must be made. One area of concern is whether or not to appoint a project director. A designated project director provides the change project with someone who is not burdened with other responsibilities. A limitation to this role is that many times the individual assumes the total accountability for the change project but has little to no line authority. In this instance, it is very difficult to actually implement a change. If a project director is selected, this individual must act more as a resource to the project team. The project team has the ultimate authority and the accountability to implement the change.

Staff nurse council chairpersons require significant support. For example, some organizations allocate a portion of a chairperson's paid time to the conduct of council's business. Other strategies include preplanning for additional coverage to staff the unit, while certain nurses attend council meetings. The support of the individual nurse is an issue that surfaces repeatedly during implementation. Each organization must find its own solution *prior to beginning implementation ac-*

tivities. Project teams usually grossly underestimate the need for this support. Not only do staff nurse participants need assistance, managers need assistance, too. Managers must be encouraged to find creative ways of funding staff to participate, including shifts in budget allocations. If left unaddressed, nurses will burn-out from too many demands and will ultimately withdraw from the project.

Planning activities must also address the process by which membership to the new nursing councils unfolds. Will members be appointed, elected, or volunteer? An effective process is to have elected representatives to councils. For some organizations, this may be too radical of a change or it may run counter to the prevailing culture. In such instances, a volunteer method may be used. However, volunteers must meet a set of predefined criteria that will assure their success in these new professional roles. The criteria for volunteer participation should be developed as part of the planning process.

The members to nursing councils should rarely, if ever, be appointed. This fosters the perception that the system is management dominated, and leaves room for membership by virtue of position rather than skill.

Another difficult issue is to determine the time frame and the format of the implementation plan. Since the plan will be used to educate individuals and groups about the direction and progress of the change, care must be taken to make it "user-friendly." Also, planning too far in advance may result in implementation steps that are inaccurate because of unknowns.

An example of an implementation plan is included in Exhibit 7-4. Steps can be delineated for each of the major councils under a shared governance structure, using this format. Note that not only are implementation steps identified but also the conceptual theme of the activity. The plan is divided into six-month segments, to allow for necessary adjustments to the plan and to give direction for evaluation activities.

In this example, project team assessments revealed that the nursing quality assurance program needed strengthening, prior to the implementation of a Quality Assurance Council under a shared governance structure. It was decided that a unit-based quality assurance program would be implemented first, while other shared governance councils were in various stages of development. Over one year was dedicated to developing and formalizing the unit-based quality assurance program, before a Nursing Quality Assurance Council was implemented.

Exhibit 7-4 Restructure to a Quality Assurance Council (Evaluation is a Professional Nursing Responsibility)

August to January 1989

- Develop unit-based program definitions
- Create unit-based committees
- Decentralize quality assurance coordination
- Redesign current quality assurance committee to include unit-based membership
- Begin in-services on unit-based quality assurance
- Determine new relationship of nursing quality assurance to hospital program

January to June 1989

- Develop subcommittee to identify Quality Assurance Council structure and processes
- Disband code committee and incident review committee
- Add code committee to critical care unit-based committee
- Add incident review reporting to Quality Assurance Coordinating Committee
- Integrate infection control practitioner into QA program
- Develop handbooks for unit-based quality assurance committees

June to January 1990

- Complete bylaws for Quality Assurance Council
- Implement Quality Assurance Council based on bylaws
- Develop conceptual subcommittee to identify the integration of credentialling and evaluation processes
- Implement a QA Coordinating Committee to direct unit-based program
- Define specialist and educator role further, in relation to unit-based quality assurance
- Continue quality assurance in services
- Develop and implement operational processes to monitor and trend quality assurance activities, including a computer program to track and trend
- Identify first departmental monitors

Planning activities were divided into six-month segments, in order to allow for the appearance of unexpected events and to promote plan flexibility. This was a useful segmentation of planning, since several events slowed implementation of a Nursing Quality Assurance Council. First, the hospital suddenly decided to implement an integrated quality assurance and utilization review program. This necessitated changes in the integration of unit-based quality assurance activities with the rest of the organization. Also, the Joint Commission on the Accreditation of Hospital Organizations (JCAHO) shifted its focus to outcome monitoring. Both changes required significant alterations of the implementation plan.

Another crucial issue central to successful implementation is the determination of where participation fits in the current nursing reward system. This is an area commonly overlooked in planning. The philosophy of participation must be decided in advance of actual implementation and communicated clearly to the nursing staff. Is participation in the council structure an expectation or is it voluntary? When and how will nurses be reimbursed for the time to participate? If the council work is deemed as important as the actual delivery of care, then appropriate decisions will be made.

NURSING COUNCIL IMPLEMENTATION

In the first year of the implementation plan, much of the activity is focused on the preparation and education of key groups. Everyone needs to understand the council structure, its membership, and the manner in which decision making will change. Potential staff nurse members will need additional education about the actual process of hospital decision-making, and where the council activity will fit within that process. This will be new information, in many cases. In one organization, a staff nurse reported that she now understood "why it took so long to get anything done." She had recognized the need to facilitate certain decisions through several professional groups before implementation. Some staff nurses will require assistance in developing effective group and leadership skills. Preparing meeting agendas, facilitating discussions, and dealing with group conflicts may not be part of the skill set of some staff nurses.

In the first year, the manager group should be identifying management development needs, in preparation for broader operational authority. In one organization, a survey of educational needs was administered to managers and used to guide education throughout implementation. Planning and financial management were at the top of the list.

The second year of implementation sees the first nursing councils emerge. It is wise to order the emergence of councils, so that there is a balance in the pace and amount of change in the organization. In the third year, the nursing organization decision making happens through the council structure. Much of the focus during this time is to identify coordinating mechanisms and adjust the structure as necessary.

Nursing Practice Council

The Nursing Practice Council commonly emerges first. It is one of the more exciting changes and also the easiest to articulate. The early work of this council is to provide the cornerstones of nursing practice for the rest of the nursing organization, through the adoption of a conceptual framework and practice standards. Early issues will arise over the ownership of policies and procedures, and the manager's role on the practice council. For example, the clinical specialist may feel threatened at first. Clinical nursing practice issues can be the predominant source of specialists influence in the organization. Predefined bylaws or operating policies will facilitate resolution of these issues.

The Nursing Practice Council must be provided with knowledge of and access to organizational resources. A planned orientation for new members, including an orientation packet, could include that information as well as role expectations.

It is important that early decision making is successful. Nursing leaders should search for problems that have a high probability of being easily solved, and refer these to the Nursing Practice Council. As the group becomes more expert, the problems addressed by the council will become more complex.

Nursing Management Council

The Nursing Management Council must emerge close to the time of the Nursing Practice Council. A strong management council is essential to the success of a councilor structure. The implementation needs of the Nursing Management Council can be seriously underestimated during planning. For example, if nursing manager authority for nursing organization decisions is not defined properly, management issues will be found in the decision-making activities of other shared governance councils. Such an error can occur when the management team lacks expertise or when top nursing administration is reluctant to define the authority boundaries of nursing management roles. In such instances, the Nursing Management Council is not making decisions. It will remain a hierarchically structured group, which comes together to share information.

This outcome puts the entire structure at risk for rejection by the nursing staff. Rejection is based upon a perception that the structure was invented in order to do "management's work." Unfortunately, this perception may be correct. Because certain management decisions are necessary to support the work of the nursing councils, management decisions will appear in these councils only if the Nursing Management Council is ineffective. If this problem does occur, a significant realignment of council responsibilities must occur, including activities to strengthen the role of the Nursing Management Council.

The effectiveness of the management council is the direct responsibility of top nursing administrators. It is not an easy task. Managers must be equally empowered through the council structure, in order to leave behind a major focus on clinical decision making.

Early council work includes the examination of nurse manager job descriptions for evidence of appropriate operational authority at all levels. First line managers expand their scope of operational responsibility as unit clinical issues are increasingly handled by the staff. The sphere of influence broadens at each administrative level. Nursing management layers may disappear. The numbers of management positions are reduced purposefully or by attrition. The nursing organization will flatten out into an open, networking environment.

The nursing administrator benefits from the improved performance of subordinates. The empowerment of the management team under shared governance allows the nursing administrator to shift from a focus on everyday operations to participation in the key strategic planning and economic activities of the whole organization. The nursing organization will be positioned for true partnership when this involvement is realized at the board level.

The implementation of the Nursing Management Council is uniquely challenging because every member functions as supervisor and as subordinate. This characteristic of Nursing Management Council members may make decision making and problem solving constrained, for fear of disagreeing with a supervisor in a public forum. Some organizations have used outside group facilitators to help deal with the authority issues posed by the implementation of a Nursing Management Council.

Nursing Quality Assurance Council

The Nursing Quality Assurance Council also has unique implementation needs, which must be identified during planning. The effectiveness of the quality assurance program and the structure of the program must be examined in light of the new council structure. Integration issues may be significant if there is a strong quality assurance program outside of nursing's purview. Decisions must also be made about the integration of performance reviews and career ladder activities into council functions. These are sensitive people issues and often require the cooperation and insight of skilled human resource experts.

Because this arena of nursing work is highly regulated, it is important that the early chairperson be an expert in the quality assurance process and the JCAHO standards. In this way, the staff nurse participants on the council will benefit from the expertise of a strong leader, and the integrity of the nursing quality assurance program will remain intact. Once the Nursing Quality Assurance Council is functioning effectively, the volume and excellence of the quality assurance studies will improve dramatically. As in all decentralized systems, the coordination of the nursing quality assurance program is central to the attainment of this outcome.

Nursing Education Council

The Nursing Education Council struggles with issues similar to those of the Nursing Quality Assurance Council. Planning must identify the implementation activities necessary for successful implementation. Nursing education activities and their budgets will become more decentralized under the shared governance structure. If the education department is presently centralized, how will this change occur? The work of implementation is more complicated if the education department does not report to nursing. In this scenario, educators are often required to maintain an institution-wide focus. The blending of this focus with the defined authority of the nursing staff is delicate work. In addition, the work of the educators and clinical nurse specialists is folded into the council functions. These individuals struggle as the locus of control for their teaching activities shifts to the council's authority. Considerable support is needed at this time, to assure successful role resolution. Not only should teachers be supported, but the council must be encouraged to keep the authority for the determination of educational needs in the nursing organization.

Nursing Executive Council

The Nursing Executive/Governance Committee emerges last. It is sometimes the outgrowth of the project team. For example, in one organization, the evolution of the governance council occurred through the transformation of a shared governance task force to a steering committee. The steering committee then became the coordinating council, with an implementation plan to become the executive council of the nursing organization. Because this council serves in an executive capacity to the council structure, the chairpersons of each major council and the nurse administrator are its members.

The delineation of bylaws must assure that the executive committee does not usurp the authority of the nursing councils. Its functions are to coordinate the structure, assure its effectiveness, and arbitrate when councils disagree. If the governance council does indeed engage in decision making which is the purview of another council, then the pyramid of hierarchy has been replicated in the council structure.

Nursing's tradition of hierarchy commonly produces an implementation error where councils and their unit-based counterparts form levels rather than lateral communication networks. Planning activities must include the identification methods to detect pyramids, if they begin to develop!

CULTURE STRATEGIES

Six to eight months should be spent in preparing an organization for the actual implementation of a new organizational structure. For example, in one hospital, the project was kicked-off with a series of all-day workshops for clinical and administrative leadership groups. The workshops identified the relationship of shared governance to the organization's past, present, and future. A reading list was prepared and copies of the articles were made available. Repeated formal presentations were made to key nursing groups. These were then followed up by informal discussion groups.

Once key nursing groups have been educated about the change, meetings begin with other key groups of professionals. The top nursing administrator continues discussions with the CEO, translating the positive outcomes of shared governance for the organization and monitoring support for the project. Repeated exchanges of information occur between nursing and other departments.

Hospital departments having significant involvement with nursing functions need special attention. For example, in one hospital, the pharmacy leadership was involved in several nursing committees where medication practices were discussed. These individuals were helped to understand the new structure and participated in defining their place within it. In another organization, the central education department needed special attention.

Those individuals responsible for organizational preparation will use the opportunity to educate to prepare the organization. Educational sessions are also opportunities to gather information about how the change is being perceived.

ANTICIPATING IMPLEMENTATION "HOTSPOTS"

Who Will Participate?

The project team must plan the actual stages of council implementation. If anticipated in advance, certain problems can be avoided during implementation. A significant problem to be addressed is the definition of who will participate in what kind of decisions.

The nursing staff of most hospitals is made up of both professional nurses and nursing support staff. Needs for support staff recognition must be balanced with the requirement for knowledgeable professional nurses to make decisions about clinical practice. At the outset of the project, a clearly identified place for support nursing staff must be created and implemented. If this does not happen, considerable dissatisfaction of these groups may be the result.

This issue has been resolved in many different ways. Some nursing organizations have established unit or clinical service quality circles that include nursing support staff. These groups work with managers to solve everyday work place problems interfering with quality care. Other organizations have included support personnel into unit-based committees that relate to the larger nursing councils. Both methods have been successful in the integration of support personnel.

The kind of decisions for which the nursing staff has authority must be carefully defined and comprehensively communicated. There must be recognition that the authority for decision making in a hospital is "shared." If pay and benefit issues are not included in the decision-making authority of the staff, this must be clearly articulated within the organization.

Timing Council Development

Another set of decisions determines how councils will actually emerge under the new shared governance structure. Which ones will emerge first? Each nursing activity is scrutinized closely. Based upon this examination, decisions can be made as to how that activity will be folded into a shared governance council's purpose and functions. Some of the functions and systems of the nursing organization are stronger than others. Councils assuming those strong functions should be allowed to emerge first. While these councils are being implemented, work can be done on the weaker systems, to ready them for council involvement.

Conceptualizing the Change

To aid in this process, all but the critical work of nursing committees should be stopped. The project team should anticipate that there may be some resistance to this step. Those committees and activities with similar themes can be grouped together, in order to explore how they may be merged into a new structure. For example, in one organization, approximately twenty-three committees were merged into five conceptual planning groups with common themes. In order to break down old identities, the groups were given numbers instead of names. They were called conceptual planning groups in order to emphasize the need to think through the change before taking action.

Each group was asked to identify the answers to the following questions:

1. What has been the work of each committee?
2. What are the likes and dislikes regarding the committee work?
3. What do you need to know about shared governance?

4. What would the work of this committee be, under a council or structure?
5. Write a purpose for a potential council, combining the activities of your committees.
6. What authority for what decisions should be vested in this council?
7. What resources will be necessary for this group to attain council status?
8. How will this council relate to other councils?

The responses of conceptual planning groups to these questions can then be shared with the shared governance project team and integrated into planning activities. In the prior example, over twenty-three committees were replaced by five councils and seven subcommittees of the larger councils. The evolution of these councils from the many nursing committees in this example is outlined in Figure 7-1.

Coordination/Integration Needs

The coordination and monitoring of implementation activities also need to be addressed during implementation. Each nursing group can be required to submit an annual report of the group's activities and progress towards implementation. The contents of such a report are outlined in Exhibit 7-5. Annual reports can be used by both the conceptual group and the nursing councils, once they have been formally introduced. The data collected can be used to evaluate progress in implementation as well as the council/committee effectiveness.

The integration of the council work must also be facilitated at the clinical and the unit level. It is here that managers translate the work of the councils to the delivery of patient care. Managers are successful to the extent that they link the work of the council to nursing practice at the bedside. When this does not happen, the shared governance councils are seen as irrelevant to patient care.

Bylaws

The implementation of shared governance structures must also be accompanied by the early development of bylaws. This, too, is the work of the project team, in collaboration with the conceptual planning

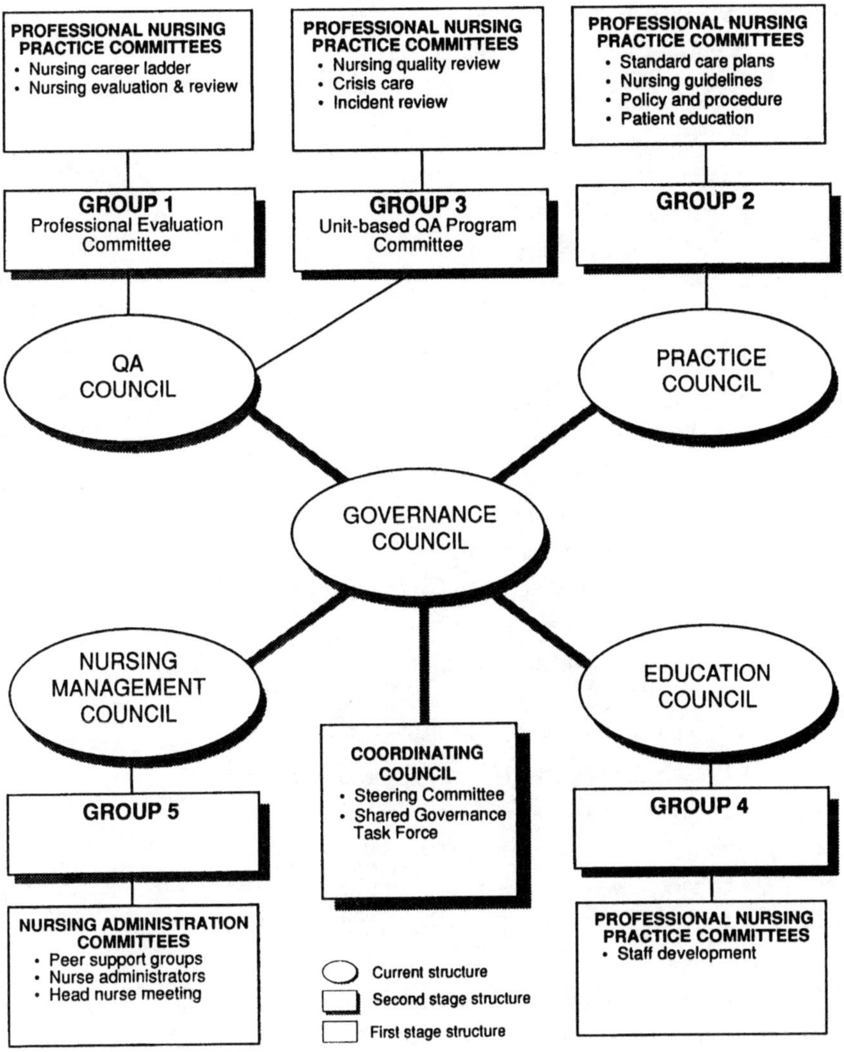

Figure 7-1 Nursing Committee Transformation to a Shared Governance Structure

groups. The absence of bylaws makes it difficult to identify the authority for decision making and the requisite operations of each council.

The initiation of bylaws is a difficult and sensitive issue for the nursing organization. At the minimum, operating policies must be developed for each group. Otherwise, there will be significant conflicts

Exhibit 7-5 Format for Nursing Committee/Council Annual Report

Major Focus of Decision Making
Activities and Outcomes Strategies
- Group membership
- Attendance

Committee/Council Effectiveness
- Cohesiveness
- Peer process
- Interaction
- Membership understanding of group function

Problem-Solving Effectiveness
- Use of resources
- Acceptance of new ideas
- Task achievement and follow-up
- Congruity of problems with Committee/Council purpose
- Preparation of members for meetings
- Degree of equal participation of members
- Ability of group to self-evaluate its work
- Evaluation of decisions for effectiveness
- Inadequate response of group/individual addressed
- Effective attention release mechanism

Leadership
- Formal
- Informal
- Future

Progress of Shared Governance Implementation Relationships
Future Goals

over authority. Council operating policies parallel bylaws, but do not have the legitimate authority of the organization vested in them by the hospital board of directors. If council operating policies do not eventually become bylaws for the nursing organization, the legitimacy of the shared governance structure is open to question.

Coordination

Finally, the actual implementation of nursing councils should be accompanied by methods for coordinating and integrating the work of the councils. For example, one organization implemented a form called an "action item request." This document could be used by an individual, a group, or a nursing council to request that a problem be acted upon. The form was completed in triplicate, with copies going to the sender, the intended council, and the nursing office. Each request was numbered. Once a solution was identified and implemented, the form was completed, returned to the sender, and filed in the nursing office. In this way, the status and volume of all decision making in the council structure could be tracked.

THE OUTCOMES OF SHARED GOVERNANCE

The decision to create a shared governance structure is a landmark decision for most nursing organizations. The successful implementation requires the commitment of strong clinical and administrative leaders. Significant resources are used during implementation. Is it worth it? The outcomes speak for themselves.

The implementation of a shared governance structure can be a powerful influence on the professional practice environment of nurses. In fact, the implementation of the decision-making structure itself has led to the development of other key components of a professional practice environment. Shared governance organizations are strongly represented in the magnet hospital follow-up studies,[33] testifying to the power of such organizations to attract and retain qualified professional nurses.

Patient care is of a high caliber in shared governance organizations. For example, some of the earliest case management systems emerged from nursing organizations that defined and gave authority to effective nursing roles. In certain shared governance organizations, patient documentation systems reflect the theory of professional nursing and are commonly integrated with the medical record of care. Joint physician-nurse committees are strong and effective in providing collaborative solutions to patient care problems. For example, in one shared governance organization, the Chief of the Medical Staff, the president-elect, and the past president meet regularly with the Nursing Executive

Council to collaborate on patient care problems. Nurses in shared governance organizations participate and have authority for their own quality assurance work. Studies are abundant, well-defined, and patient care incidents have been described as declining in number. All of these activities combine to assure the cost-effective provision of patient care.

The financial effectiveness of shared governance structures has been reported in the literature. Salary savings from the reduction in management positions offset the increased costs associated with meetings. The cost of meeting time to the organization for one year's time was less than 1.5% of the total budgeted full-time equivalents for the nursing organization.[34]

Most significantly, the power of the structure to stimulate clinical nursing leadership is awesome. This outcome alone makes membership in a shared governance organization a vital, worthwhile, and professionally satisfying experience. It is well worth the trials, tribulations, and resource expenditures that accompany successful implementation.

NOTES

1. Porter-O'Grady, T. and Finnigan, S. (1984). *Shared Governance for Nursing.* Gaithersburg, MD: Aspen Publishers, Inc.
2. American Academy of Nursing. (1983). *Magnet Hospitals: Attraction and Retention of Professional Nurses.* Kansas City, MO: American Nurses Association.
3. Institute of Medicine. (1982). *The Study of Nursing and Nursing Education.* Washington, DC: National Academy of Sciences.
4. National Commission on Nursing. (1982). *Summary Report and Recommendations.* Chicago: American Hospital Association.
5. Sashkin, M. (1984). Participative management in an ethical imperative. *Organizational Behavior,* 12(2), 5–21.
6. Sashkin, M. (1986). Participative management remains an ethical imperative. *Organizational Behavior,* 14(2), 62–75.
7. Schwartz, G. and Comstock, V. (1979). One firm's experiences with quality circles. *Quality Progress,* 12(9), 14–16.
8. Locke, E.A. and Lathom, G. (1984). *Goal Setting—A Motivational Technique that Works.* Englewood Cliffs, NJ: Prentice-Hall.
9. Schwartz, G. and Comstock, V. (1979). One firm's experiences with quality circles. *Quality Progress,* 12(9), 14–16.
10. Schwartz, R.H. (1990). Nurse decision-making influence. *Journal of Nursing Administration,* 29(16), 35–39.

11. Miller, K. and Mange, P. (1986). Participation, satisfaction and productivity. A meta-analytic review. *Academy of Management Journal,* 29(4), 727–753.
12. Gmeldi, W.H. and Misken, V.D. (1986). The lost art of high productivity. *Personnel,* 63(94), 34–38.
13. Sashkin, M. (1986), p. 60.
14. Wagner, J.C. and Gooding, R.Z. (1987). Shared influence and organizational behavior. A meta-analysis of situational variables expected to moderate participation outcome relationships. *Academy of Management Journal,* 30(93), 524–541.
15. Abell, P. (1979). Hierarchy and democratic authority. In T.R. Burns, L.E. Karlson and V. Rus, *Work and Power.* Beverly Hills: Sage Publications, pp. 141–171.
16. Ibid., pp. 161–169.
17. Porter-O'Grady, T. (1986). *Creative Nursing Administration.* Gaithersburg, MD: Aspen Publishers, Inc., pp. 169–194.
18. Porter-O'Grady, T. and Finnigan, S. (1984), pp. 29–35.
19. Porter-O'Grady, T. (1986), pp. 27–51.
20. Miller, L.M. (1984). *American Spirit.* New York: Warner Books, p. XVI.
21. Peters, T. and Austin, N. (1985). *A Passion For Excellence.* New York: Random House.
22. Ibid., pp. 217–219.
23. Ibid., p. 219.
24. Bass, B. (1984). *Leadership and Performance Beyond Expectations.* New York: The Free Press.
25. Porter-O'Grady, T. (1986), pp. 34–36.
26. Jackson, B. (1989). Ownership imbalance. *Journal of Nursing Administration,* 9(9), pp. 4–5.
27. Porter-O'Grady, T. and Finnigan, S. (1984), pp. 36–41.
28. Naisbett, J. and Auburdene, P. (1985). *Re-inventing the Corporation.* New York: Warner Books, pp. 44–51.
29. McDonagh, K.J., Rhondes, B., Sharbey, K., and Goodrae, J.H. (1989). Shared governance at St. Joseph's Hospital of Atlanta: A mature professional practice model. *Nursing Administration Quarterly,* 13(4), pp. 17–29.
30. Ibid., p. 21.
31. Porter-O'Grady, T. (1991). A nurse on the board. *Journal of Nursing Administration,* 21(1), 40–46.
32. Porter-O'Grady, T. and Finnegan, S. (1984).
33. Kramer, M. and Schmalenberg, C. (1988), Magnet hospitals: Part I: Institutions of excellence. *Journal of Nursing Administration,* 18(1), 13–24.
34. Jenkins, J. (1988), A nursing governance and practice model: What are the costs? *Nursing Economics,* 6(6), p. 309.

CHAPTER 8

Delivery System Redesign—Making It Worth Your While

Carol Hatler and Kathy Malloch

This chapter focuses on the implementation and evaluation of a delivery system redesign. This restructuring activity took place in a midsized community hospital in the Southwest between early 1988 and early 1991. Elements of this change included implementation of differentiated RN practice and institution of an unlicensed caregiver for non-nursing tasks on two pilot units. The following are described: 1) items and rationale for evaluation methods, 2) implementation of the delivery system changes, and 3) recommendations regarding the role of project evaluator.

FACTORS MANDATING REDESIGN AND PROJECT EVALUATION

Health care organizations, like other open systems, respond to environmental stressors. Within the current health care arena, these environmental stressors include decreased financial resources, increased competition for patients, decreased human resources, new technologies, patient demographic changes, a shift from inpatient to outpatient care settings and concomitant patient care issues. These stressors were felt within the health care organization described in this chapter as a RN vacancy rate of 30% and increased use of per diem nursing staff. Clearly organizational changes were needed to address these issues and the health care organization adapted by restructuring patient care delivery.

In determining the value of organizational changes, the project team gave considerable thought to the purposes for and outcomes of restructuring activities. The goal of the evaluation activities for this project was an effective and efficient delivery system that maintained patient care quality. In addition, the professional nurses involved in the project believed that systematic evaluation of the change process and outcomes was essential. Nurses know that providing nursing care, without identifying treatment goals, often results in wasted time, effort, and supplies. In the same manner, implementing organizational changes without determining the goals of the change process can also produce inappropriate resource use. Within today's resource-driven market, it was mandatory that evaluation of delivery system redesign occur in a logical manner.

LIMITATIONS TO CONTEMPORARY EVALUATION PRACTICES

Little empirical evidence exists regarding criteria for evaluating organizational restructuring. Within the literature, numerous anecdotal accounts appear describing evaluation elements and processes.[1,2,3] However, little systematic examination of these evaluation components has been reported. Narratives of projects can benefit those considering organizational change ("We did it this way and this is how it worked"). Narratives are limited, however, because there is rarely assurance that the implemented change could be replicated. How can we know if the methods used in one health care organization, which produced certain results, would also work in a different organization or environment?

Nursing organizations implementing new structures should engage in deliberative identification of both restructuring goals and outcomes along with validated tools for measurement of critical elements of those goals. This process permits a broader application of results. An additional savings can result from identifying specific project outcomes, rather than relying on individuals' judgments about the "goodness" of the outcomes.[4] Nursing leaders must consider the purposes and outcomes for restructuring activities as the first step in delivery system changes. These, then, will drive the selection of measurable objectives.

Multiple Organizational Purposes

The complexity of today's health care organizations makes the evaluation of delivery system changes particularly challenging. Campbell (1977)[5] suggested that the multiple purposes of modern organizations and the variety of perspectives from which to view each organization's performance constituted a significant barrier to adequate evaluation. In determining performance measures, multiple "users" of the health care organization must be considered. Internal organization users (caregivers, managers, administrators) tend to rely on process and fiscal criteria when evaluating performance. External users (consumers, payors), on the other hand, focus on outcomes and perceptions.[6] Therefore, a variety of performance measures are more likely to provide nursing organizations with a sound basis upon which to evaluate new structure implementation. Those considering delivery system redesign must determine which users' needs will be met by the new system. Performance measures can then be selected with these users in mind.

Timing and Sampling

The timing of data collection poses additional challenges to accurate restructuring evaluation. For health care organizations, the necessity of obtaining information without interrupting the processes of the system produces unique difficulties.[7] It would be inappropriate to suspend or curtail patient care activities in order to collect evaluative information. As a result, arbitrary data elements and data collection times are often selected.

A "hit or miss" approach to the sampling of evaluation elements can prove hazardous. Results may or may not represent a true picture of the organization. For example, consider that measures of nurses' job satisfaction differ, depending on staffing levels and patient care acuity. Similarly, financial results vary for health care organizations depending on patient mix and physician practice patterns. Differences in financial information may also appear, depending on how financial reports are constructed and distributed. Evaluating delivery system changes based on single criteria sets can lead to decisions that do not accurately predict future trends. The demands of consumers, caregivers, administrators, and the environment, therefore, must be included in evaluation of organizational change.

A SYSTEMS FRAMEWORK FOR EVALUATION

By factoring in the diverse needs of users, evaluation design and implementation follows a "multiple constituency approach."[8] Sampling from multiple users of the organization reflects a holistic, systems approach to thinking about evaluation. This systems thinking facilitates understanding of complex phenomena such as organizational behavior. When the evaluation plan is designed within a systems theory framework, the results are more credible.

By sampling from multiple sources, opposition to change can be reduced. Incomplete evaluation processes and outcomes inadequately describe project achievement. The new structure is then open to criticism. Consider the following scenario:

> A large metropolitan health care organization contracted with an independent consulting firm to evaluate its cost-per-case operations. The consulting firm focused on the number and types of patients the organization admitted as well as the reimbursement for each of these patient types. The results of the evaluation met with vigorous objections from caregivers and managers. These caregivers and managers pointed out that the evaluation methods did not include significant factors which impacted costs. These objections lead to skepticism about the evaluation methods and results.
>
> As a result, little change occurred within the organization. Had the consulting firm taken a systems approach to the project, caregivers and managers would have been polled regarding their perspectives on the cost-per-case issue. From these discussions, then, would have come broader evaluation methods and a credible solution which promoted change.

Systems Theory and Evaluation

Use of a systems theory conceptual framework is crucial to evaluation planning since it makes it easier to

- identify essential properties of the new structure
- analyze structure components and predict their relationships
- identify connections between seemingly unrelated elements and occurrences[9,10]

The application of systems theory principles to evaluation within organizations allows for the explanation and prediction of occurrences during the implementation of new nursing structures.

Systems theory identifies a system as a bounded set of interrelated units that exist in a given environment. A distinctive characteristic of a system is that the dynamic composite equates to more than simply a sum of the component parts. The interaction between components produces a more potent entity when viewed as a whole. This emphasis on totality of the system suggests that the individual components of the system can be understood only in relation to the whole. When viewing health care organizations as a system, the evaluation of new nursing structures must be examined within the context of the whole organization.

For example, the processes and actions involved in the initial assessment for a hospitalized individual reflect a systems approach. The actions of business office personnel, laboratory and radiologic technicians, and health care providers produce a composite of information. The information from all departments makes up a more meaningful total picture of the individual's condition than do isolated actions and bits of information.

The Evaluation of Delivery Systems and Systems Thinking

Additional characteristics of a system are those boundaries which separate internal and external environments. The boundaries of health care organizations exist both physically and conceptually. In an open system, such as a health care organization, each component of the system exchanges energy (e.g., information and resources) across and within its boundaries. In this way, change in a particular portion of the system affects the total system and each of its components.[12] In a health care organization patient care delivery changes influence other organizational processes. Affected processes include allocation of salaries, level at which decision making occurs, and staffing patterns. Evaluating a new patient care delivery system must take into account the interrelationship of organizational units and processes.

Figure 8-1 illustrates some of the organizational variables influenced by changes in the delivery system. Both relationships and processes of patient care are affected by redesign activities. The relationships between individual nurses and between nurses and ancillary support staff will be altered by delivery system changes.

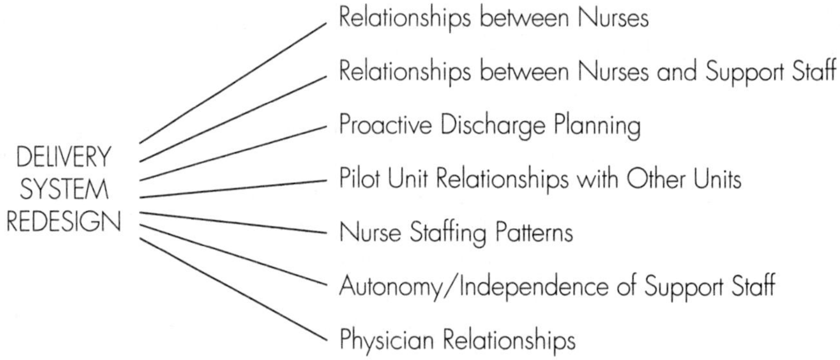

Fig 8.1 Some Organizational Variables Influenced by Delivery System Redesign

Within previous delivery systems, nurses may have functioned as peers with every nurse responsible for the same kinds of tasks and outcomes. With some delivery system changes, however, nurses' responsibilities change. Nurses must develop collegial rather than peer relationships. Nurse staffing patterns must change to reflect these different responsibilities.

Altered nursing responsibilities, including proactive care and discharge planning, necessitate changes in patterns of staffing and workflow for ancillary support departments. Ancillary staff members (physical therapists, social workers, dietitians) frequently schedule patient treatments based on departmental patterns. New delivery systems, however, focus on activities that facilitate patient movement through the system. As a result of this patient focus, it is necessary for ancillary departments to change their patterns. With alterations in the autonomy of ancillary staff come changes in relationships and communications with nurses.

DEFINING THE EVALUATION PROJECT

Using a systems approach, the project planning and evaluation team identified essential elements that would indicate attainment of restructuring project goals. The goals of this project were similar to those identified by Brett and Tonges (1990).[13] Specifically, project goals included the implementation of a delivery system that maintained and/or improved:

- nurses' job satisfaction and retention (including position vacancies and turnover)
- quality of patient care as evidenced by nurses' compliance with process indicators and decreased patient complications, patient satisfaction with care, and length of stay data relating to the top five DRGs on the units' populations
- the cost-effectiveness of care delivery including hours per patient day, overtime costs, supplemental agency nurse costs, salary cost per patient day, and paid dollars per full-time equivalent

By measuring these concepts, outcomes of the new delivery system can be documented. Measures and rationale for each of the evaluation elements are described separately.

Nurse Job Satisfaction

Human resources are the most valuable asset possessed by any health care organization. In general, the less an organization alienates its personnel, the more efficient it becomes.[14] Efforts aimed at retaining personnel benefit the organization in many ways. Replacement costs for a single RN, in terms of recruitment and orientation, range from $2000 to $3000.[15] It makes sense that those health care organizations requiring fewer dollars to replace nurses will fare better financially. Factors influencing nurses' work satisfaction include work scheduling, a lack of stimulating work, and overall life satisfaction. In addition, the presence of alternative career opportunities and certain demographic characteristics influence nurses' work satisfaction. Investigators[16,17] have identified overall job satisfaction as a major predictor of turnover intention. By identifying and focusing on critical elements of nurses' work satisfaction, health care organizations can more readily retain professional nurses.

The complex nature of work satisfaction and motivation prompted the project team to select tools that sampled a variety of aspects relating to nurse satisfaction. A tool originated by Slavitt, et al (1978)[18] and modified by Hinshaw and Atwood (1987)[19] was chosen. This tool contained subscales to measure nurses' satisfaction with pay, professional status, group cohesion/interaction, administration, and task requirements—areas critical to the organizational environment. Each tool had demonstrated acceptable validity and reliability (r=.75 and r=.67, respectively). In addition, RN vacancy and turnover rates indicated nurse satisfaction with the organization.

Quality of Care

To obtain information from multiple users of the delivery system and to gain a more complete picture of functional changes, quality of care elements must be evaluated. The usefulness of Quality Assurance/ Quality Resource Management (QA/QRM) outcomes is influenced by a number of factors. These factors include the structure of the QA/QRM department and process, the politics of QA/QRM information flow within the organization, the performance of those responsible for synthesizing QA data, and the adequacy of the data collection system.

The Quality Assurance/Quality Resource Management (QA/QRM) program of a health care organization provides the mechanism by which consumers, payors, and regulatory agencies are assured of ongoing care improvement. Donabedian (1980)[20] identified characteristics of effective quality assurance programs. These characteristics include a balance of activities between those focused on preserving health and preventing harm with those activities that focus on avoiding useless care. The effectiveness of a health care organization's QA/QRM is influenced by its structure. Most frequently the QA/QRM program is structured either centrally or decentralized with a unit-based approach.

Regardless of structure, the active involvement of staff nurses in these processes is essential. Formella and Schroeder (1984)[21] suggest that when the QA/QRM process involves practicing nurses, patient care problems can be detected and solved in a timely manner. In this way, QA/QRM activities reduce organizational liability and improve patient care.

By demonstrating a commitment to professional nursing by supporting QA/QRM activities, a health care organization can contribute to nursing satisfaction and retention. There is a link between practice-based QA/QRM activities and nursing accountability and autonomy.[22,23] By enhancing nurses' control of practice in this way, organizations retain professional nurses.

Specific QA/QRM elements used to evaluate the differentiated practice project included number and type (falls, medication errors, skin breakdown) of patient incidents. Since the project focused on redesign of nursing roles, it was reasoned that these occurrences reflected patient outcomes under nurses' control.

Initially information about these QA/QRM elements was easily obtained from existing reports. Difficulties arose, however, in interpreting the information. Current records provided no mechanism to indicate whether or not patients required further treatment as a result of the incident. Consequently, nurse managers are unable to evaluate these incidents in terms of severity. Only the number of items can be evaluated and this yields incomplete information about the quality of care.

Financial Evaluation Elements

Traditionally, nonprofit health care organizations have overlooked the cost-benefit analysis of proposed organizational changes. Health care providers are reluctant to base decisions on criteria other than patient need. Indeed, decisions based on resource use are viewed by many in nonprofit health care organizations as unethical and uncaring. The current fiscal realities of health care mandate evaluation of organizational changes in terms of their impact on operating costs.

Organizational efforts to reduce losses and maximize reimbursement have generated financial reports detailing direct and indirect costs and revenue. The format and timing of this information, however, poses difficulties when evaluating restructuring activities. Reports such as occupancy rates, average length of stay, capital expense and depreciation, and average revenue by patient type allow analysis of trends over time. Reports like these most often appear four to six weeks after the actual occurrences. This delayed timing hampers timely analysis and problem solving. In addition, the available pieces of an organization's financial picture are often fragmented to the extent that considerable effort is needed to synthesize a complete view.

The difficulties described in obtaining accurate and timely information led the project team to select direct salary costs as the financial criteria included in project evaluation. Since the new delivery system involved changes in caregiver type and function, salary costs would reasonably be the most sensitive financial indicator of change. Financial goals of the project included reduction of overtime costs and reduction of per diem salary costs. These results were expected from more appropriate use of RNs through role differentiation and from delegation of non-nursing tasks to an unlicensed unit aid.

IMPLEMENTATION OF THE CHANGE

The Setting

Maryvale Samaritan Medical Center (MSMC) is a 256-bed facility in Phoenix, Arizona. In the fall of 1987, the impact of environmental stressors was perceived to be at a critical level. The nursing shortage had a severe impact on the utilization of supplemental agency nurses, nurse satisfaction, turnover, recruitment, and retention. At the same time, the realities of the prospective payment system had adversely affected the expense/reimbursement ratio. Current literature was replete with reports of the "state of the health care system" and the prevalent discrepancy in matching patient care needs with fiscal and manpower resources.

MSMC leadership encourages critical thinking, and views obstacles as opportunities for growth and as a means to improve the future of health care. Active staff participation is an important component in the MSMC culture. MSMC leaders actively attempt to inspire and facilitate staff in the analysis and synthesis of information and to address issues and resolve conflict. Yet, when faced with multiple system stressors, these leaders struggled with the wisdom of major system upheaval in the face of the nursing shortage. The dilemma of "do nothing" or "do something, even if it is wrong" was discussed at length.

Planning for Change

The decision was made to begin with an analysis of the state of the current patient care delivery system. From this initial assessment would then come the decision about whether to and in what manner to alter the current system. Staff and managers from two medical/surgical units volunteered to participate in the discussions. These two units represented differing patient populations and nursing resources. One unit was a 32-bed general surgical unit with patients who were acutely ill and had relatively short lengths of stay. The manager had recruited and retained a stable nursing staff. Turnover was low and morale was generally good. The second unit was a 32-bed general medical unit with a patient population of chronically ill individuals experiencing an acute episode. The manager was able to recruit many excellent nurses, but turnover was high, use of supplemental agency nurses was increasing, and morale was declining.

To begin the discussion, the conventional strategic planning SWOT outline was used. The SWOT framework focused on identification of existing programs and services and future possibilities. The four categories in this framework include: internal strengths (S) of the organization, internal weaknesses (W) of the organization, external opportunities (O), and external threats (T) as they relate to the topic at hand. Using the SWOT analysis is a good example for staff that project planning time is valued and that input from all participants is recognized. Information from this analysis provided the basis for selecting priorities and strategies.

In preparation for the SWOT sessions, participants were given information related to two important concepts: change theory and value systems of nonprofit organizations. Information about change theory assisted participants in dealing constructively with the human emotions associated with organizational analysis and change. Those interested in delivery system redesign may find an article by Perlman and Takacs[24] a useful tool to share with project participants. This article provides a comprehensive summary of anticipated behaviors and emotions related to change. In addition, the authors suggest strategies to facilitate the change process.

The concept of value systems of the nonprofit organization was also introduced. Rarely do organizations, such as hospitals, examine their value system history in light of its nonprofit status and relate this to the current state of affairs. Nonprofit organizations are prone to consider everything they do to be righteous and moral and to serve a cause. Nonprofit organizations, instead, need to use the discipline of critical analysis and resource-based priority setting as part of system evaluation. Once priorities are acknowledged, innovation is possible. This process begins with the recognition that change is not a threat; it is an opportunity.[25]

An integrated planning approach was used. All staff members (2 managers, 36 registered nurses, 2 LPNs, 2 nursing assistants, and 6 unit secretaries) were invited to participate in the SWOT discussions. Several sessions were held to facilitate maximum participation. Information collected from these sessions is shown in Exhibit 8-1.

Staff members reviewed all information. It was determined that a change in our nursing care delivery system was needed. The total patient care model that had been in place was inoperable, due to a shortage of RNs. After reviewing the strengths and weaknesses of vari-

Exhibit 8-1 Analysis of Organization

Strengths

1. MSMC leadership is futuristic, supportive of change, and willing to try new projects.
2. Core nursing staff are knowledgeable and committed to the organization.
3. Good reputation for quality patient care.
4. Clinical ladder program in place.
5. Flexible scheduling is encouraged.

Weaknesses

1. Shortage of qualified nurses; vacancies are increasing.
2. Nurses are overworked, dissatisfied, and underpaid.
3. New graduates are not adequately prepared.
4. Too many non-nursing tasks; too much documentation.
5. Educational preparation is not recognized at the bedside.
6. Patient classification system fails to capture what nurses really do.
7. Nurses have minimal delegation skills.

Opportunities

1. Recruit more nurses.
2. Become role model for professional practice (external recognition).
3. Strengthen affiliation with local colleges of nursing.
4. Improve collaborative care planning.
5. Encourage professional growth and development.
6. Provide information to improve patient classification system.

Threats

1. National nursing shortage; excessive use of registry nurses.
2. Decreasing third-party reimbursement.
3. Increasing regulation, e.g., HSAG.
4. Increasing competition for patients.
5. Decreasing recruitment due to internal system changes.
6. Sabotage, resistance to change.

ous methods of patient care delivery, differentiated RN practice was the approach selected in our facility to begin the process of system redesign.[26]

Overall goal identification was designed to correct weaknesses and to capitalize on opportunities. Specifically, staff nurses identified the following goals:

- Attract sufficient qualified caregivers.
- Create an environment to retain staff and achieve quality patient care.
- Focus on quality within available resources.
- Develop a framework to recognize nurses' academic preparation and clinical experience.
- Maximize commitment to excellence.

Once goals were identified, efforts focused on selection of evaluation criteria. Identification of a comprehensive criteria set that would capture the total impact on the organization was, at best, like nailing Jello to the wall. The tendency to evaluate only specific parts of the system, rather than the whole, was difficult to overcome. Other internal project evaluations included nurse turnover data, patient incidents, overtime costs, DRG costs, and FTE costs. Seldom had these been woven into an assessment of the "dynamic whole" of the delivery system.

A comprehensive group of evaluation criteria to represent elements important to internal and external users was preferred by the project team. This comprehensive information was not available, however, due to unavailable or inconsistent information sources. The final evaluation criteria were selected to best represent the delivery system components. Data for the elements selected was readily available and easily attainable. Baseline information regarding nurses' work satisfaction was obtained before discussions about system redesign began. The criteria selected (see Exhibit 8-2) included three broad categories: nurse-related data, patient-related data, and fiscal data.

Project Implementation

To begin the process of role differentiation, informational meetings were held to describe rationale for the project. Once again, multiple sessions were offered to gain maximum participation. At the completion of these sessions, it was readily apparent that enthusiasm for the project

Exhibit 8-2 Project Evaluation Elements

Patient-Related Data

- Length of stay of the top 5 DRGs of the units' populations
- Complications—medication errors, falls, nosocomial infections
- Patient satisfaction with care

Nurse-Related Data

- Work satisfaction
- Retention
- Position vacancies
- Turnover
- Compliance with use of the nursing process and discharge planning
- Participant profile information including educational preparation, length of time in nursing, age, etc.

Fiscal Data

- Hours per patient day (HPPD)
- Overtime costs
- Paid dollars per full-time equivalent (FTE)
- Supplemental agency nurse costs
- Salary cost per patient day

varied widely. A core group of nurses actively expressed interest and commitment in determining future nursing practice roles. Interested nurses continued their participation/commitment in spite of the project's uncertain outcome. Other nurses chose to remain passive and adopted a "wait and see" attitude. These individuals were folded into the project activities after initial project work had begun.

Prior to role selection, the need to select position titles was addressed. Title selection for the two roles was difficult and emotional because of the potential for disrupting the interpersonal relationships between nurses. The roles were mutually valued and position titles needed to reflect both actual roles and their value. Eventually, the titles of Case Manager and Case Associate were selected. Once titles were identified, individual role selection began.

Role selection in this transitional model was based on an individualized assessment of each nurse. With the assistance of a doctorally prepared nurse with expertise in role differentiation, each nurse selected the role most consistent with his or her knowledge, skill, and motivation, regardless of formal educational preparation or years of experience. This individual provided a valuable service in the early phases of the project.

During the role selection process and review of the two roles, nurses were able to identify many activities routinely performed that did not require the knowledge and skill of either a Case Manager or a Case Associate. In conjunction with managers, staff RNs developed a position description for a unit assistant, who would have no direct patient care responsibilities. With the help of this unit assistant, RNs can be used more effectively for activities and judgments that truly require their knowledge and skill. With RN roles defined and non-patient care activities reassigned, nurse managers were able to modify traditional patient assignments to more nearly match patient needs with staff resources. By incorporating this unit assistant role, workplace stressors could be significantly reduced and the delivery system changes were perceived as less disruptive.

Ongoing support and clarification of the new roles is, perhaps, the most critical component of role differentiation. Progress in role differentiation is directly related to the amount of time spent with each nurse in reviewing his or her practice level as compared to the chosen role. Typically, this responsibility rests with the manager. During the early stages of the project, weekly reviews were desired, but rarely possible due to managers' time constraints and staff availability. In addition, the educational preparation of the nurse managers was largely based on management theory rather than advanced nursing theory. This educational deficit made it difficult for the managers to articulate the processes and information to staff to facilitate appropriate role selection. The assistance of other nurses with expertise in role differentiation contributed significantly to progress. In the ideal situation with funding available, a dedicated project director would have helped overcome some of the obstacles. A dedicated project director would have provided resources to nurse managers and furnished coordination of restructuring efforts.

This project was internally funded and staff members provided support using a task force structure to address issues identified by nurses. These ongoing issues include:

- appropriate ratios of Case Managers/Case Associates/assistive personnel
- patient assignments to represent the Case Manager/Case Associate knowledge and skill level
- salary differentiation
- student assignments based on practice role and educational program

The nursing administrator responsible for the clinical service assumed leadership of this project. Project planning and implementation duties were taken on in addition to this individual's administrative responsibilities. The magnitude and complexity of these issues were addressed and managed without additional staff through the work of educators and the organization's nurse researcher. These individuals supported project implementation through educational presentations and intervention with staff members. Additional leadership of a project director would have facilitated progress, the timeliness of data analysis and communication of results to managers and staff.

IMPLEMENTATION OF A PROJECT EVALUATOR ROLE

The educational preparation of nurses includes little content relating to project or systems evaluation. In addition, nurses have few employment opportunities to participate in evaluation other than that of individual patient care. For these reasons, the individual faced with the opportunity to act as a project evaluator may have few resources available to draw upon. A well-designed restructuring project contains clear, measurable objects. Few sources, however, describe the "how" of project evaluation. A first-time project evaluator, then, must decide how to proceed and determine what resources exist within the health care organization.

Challenges to implementing the role of evaluator lie within three major areas.

1. assessing administrative support
2. gaining cooperation from managers and staff

3. acquiring resources for evaluation implementation

Each of these areas is essential for successful role implementation.

Administrative Support

The importance of administrative support for the project evaluator cannot be overemphasized. While project evaluation and evaluator role implementation can occur without strong administrative support, the process and outcomes of evaluation will be considerably impaired. Nursing administrators set the tone for nursing organizations. The direct and indirect power of the nursing administrator makes project implementation and evaluation difficult or easy, depending on this individual's support or opposition. Assessment of the degree of project and individual support from the nursing administrator, therefore, is crucial for those considering taking on an evaluator role. It is through administrative support that the evaluator gains credibility and cooperation of managers and staff.

How do you know if you are supported by your administrator? Administrative support contains both public and private components. Public behaviors of support include: repeated verbalization of importance of the project at organizational meetings, attendance at and participation in project planning meetings, regular inclusion of project update on organizational meeting agendas and celebration of even minor project accomplishments. Supportive behavior that is conveyed privately includes: regularly scheduled one-on-one meetings with the project evaluator, participating with the project evaluator in problem solving related to evaluation, and assisting the project evaluator to reprioritize workload demands needed.

Administrative assistance with reprioritizing workload is an essential element of support. Often, those who assume evaluator roles are expected to accomplish their new tasks in addition to all the other roles and responsibilities they have always been assigned. Multiple role expectations can lead to frustration and discouragement, since responsibility for many functions leaves the project evaluator unable to devote the time needed to any one single issue. In addition, others in the organization may continue to expect the "usual" amount and type of work from the project evaluator. When the evaluator's usual work is delayed, altered or omitted as a result of project responsibilities, other organization members may become hostile or resentful. These responses can delay or obstruct project implementation or evaluation.

Gaining Cooperation

The implementation of a delivery system redesign occurs most smoothly when organization members understand the proposed changes and then cooperate to make them happen. In order to assure cooperation from nursing managers and staff, the project evaluator must address communication, political, and action issues.

The communication of evaluation data as an opportunity for growth rather than as criticism facilitates organizational change. If this perception does not exist, dissemination of data analysis results will seem threatening to some managers and staff. For example, nurses' responses to work satisfaction questionnaires may indicate dissatisfaction with management practices. If this information were widely broadcast, or if data were reported in such a way that individuals could be identified, conflict within the organization may occur. This perception of threat could hamper the achievement of project goals and delay project evaluation. By assuring managers and staff that confidentiality will be maintained throughout the evaluation, the project evaluator can gain cooperation and proceed more easily.

Repeated information giving about all aspects of the project can often facilitate cooperation among participants. By informing people before change or measurement takes place, the project evaluator builds an atmosphere of trust. This trust relationship produces more complete evaluation data, since individuals feel comfortable telling the evaluator about concerns that could affect data results.

The project evaluator should not, however, expect cooperation from all managers or staff nurses. In every organization there are individuals for whom any change is threatening or whose need to control outweighs all others. Few strategies are likely to prove successful in gaining cooperation from such people. The most efficient use of the project evaluator's time is to discuss the resistant behavior with the individual's supervisor. The supervisor is then the person responsible for eliciting cooperation.

The organization's political climate influences the process of obtaining information. Information forms the currency of organizational power. That is, organizational members who possess considerable information related to organizational processes or outcomes may readily use this information to influence others. Those who use information as power are often unwilling to give it up, especially if doing so would undermine their power base. Project evaluators should carefully note powerful individuals in the organization and formulate strategies to incorporate these people in project implementation and evaluation. This can often be accomplished by including the individuals in planning groups. An additional strategy that facilitates cooperation is to present ideas to powerful individuals for their reactions or responses. By altering plans or processes to incorporate individuals' suggestions, the project evaluator may gain their cooperation and promote project outcomes and evaluation.

Taking Your Time

Nurses tend to focus on action, rather than thoughtful planning. This is often expressed as a "do something" response from managers and staff and an impatience with time spent in planning and evaluation. After all, the need for change has already been identified, so "let's get on with it." Possible reasons for this action orientation include a requirement for a future orientation, the undervaluing of "thinking" work and unfamiliarity with evaluation methods.

This action orientation can hamper project evaluation. Spending too little time on planning evaluation elements and methods can produce incomplete and/or inaccurate data. This erroneous data leads to inaccurate conclusions. The project evaluator must stress that the time involved in project planning and evaluation reduces project costs in the long run.

Acquiring Evaluation Resources

Following the identification of project outcomes, the specification of information needs, data analysis and reporting format require detailed consideration and development. Specifically, determination must be made about whether needed information is already available or whether different measurement tools should be identified or developed. Often the information existing within an organization is not in an easily accessed format. For example, the financial information about costs of delivering care is seldom integrated with the patient acuity system in use. Costs for individual patient conditions would be meaningless, without some matching of that information with patient care requirements. This type of information needs reformatting to allow users to make appropriate judgments about the impact of delivery system changes on the costs of care.

Additional resources required for adequate evaluation include those external to the organization. Human resources in the form of experts in clinical areas and program evaluation can assist the project evaluator. Networking with university faculty and people in other facilities who have completed similar projects proves helpful to a new project evaluator. These individuals can suggest methods, alternatives or reinforce the project evaluator's plans, thereby strengthening the entire redesign project.

Many universities maintain a listing of research or practice interests of faculty members. Connecting faculty with expertise and interest in the same areas as those of the redesign project can help the project evaluator and the faculty member. Examining literature with an eye to authors of helpful articles provides another source of external experts. Most authors are delighted to discuss their work and can provide valuable insight into methods to use and pitfalls to avoid in similar projects.

If statistical techniques are used to analyze data, consultation with an expert in this area can also be helpful. Consultation regarding the type and format of data included in project evaluation often makes analysis easier. By helping to determine beforehand the data analysis goals and the type of information needed, a statistical consultant can save time and gain credibility for the project evaluator. For example, identification of a complete set of evaluation items before the project begins allows the project evaluator to collect all the necessary data in a timely way. If this identification process does not take place, the evaluator may need to repeat data gathering activities.

In the area of statistical analysis for project evaluation, consideration must be given to availability of computer hardware and software and expertise in using these. If project outcomes call for data analysis that allows comparison or prediction of future trends, sophisticated computer equipment and expertise can prove valuable. Examples of suggested data analysis techniques are included in Exhibit 8-3.

CONCLUSION

Nursing organizations have evolved in a way that makes cost-effective practice mandatory. Within the current resource-driven health care market, we can no longer afford the luxury of making decisions without a substantive basis for change. Changes that involve people especially

Exhibit 8-3 Suggested Data Analysis Techniques for Use with Delivery System Redesign Evaluation

Chi Square

Example: Comparison of Type of Patient Complications by Type of Caregiver

ADN Med	ADN Falls	ADN Infections
Dip Med	Dip Falls	Dip Infections
BS Med	BS Falls	BS Infections

ADN=Associate Degree preparation | Dip=Diploma preparation | BS=Bachelors' preparation

Med=Medication errors | Falls=Patient falls | Infection=Nosocomial infections

Analysis of Variance

Example: Comparison of Single Variables Over Time

Dependent Variable		*Independent Variable*
Nurse Satisfaction, 1990		Nurse Satisfaction, 1988
	or	
Patient Complications 1990		Patient Complications 1988

Multiple Regression

Example: Prediction of Patient Complications by Fiscal Variables

Dependent Variable	*Independent Variables*
Number of Patient Complications	Hours per patient day Salary $ per patient day

require sound, objective rationale. By planning delivery system redesign and project evaluation proactively, nursing leaders can assist nursing organizations to truly thrive, rather than merely survive in these chaotic times.

NOTES

1. Fosbinder, D. (1986). Nursing costs/DRG: A patient classification system and comparative study. *JONA,* 16(11), 18–23.
2. Seitz, C.H. and Edwardson, S.R. (1987). Nurse care costs for stroke patients in a rehabilitation setting. *JONA,* 17(6), 17–22.
3. Neidlinger, S.H., Scroggins, K., and Kennedy, L. (1987). Cost evaluation of discharge planning for hospitalized elderly. *Nurs Econ,* 5(5), 225–230.
4. Churchman, C.W. (1968). *The Systems Approach.* New York: Dell Publishing Co., Inc.
5. Campbell, J.P. (1977). On the nature of organizational effectiveness. In *New Perspectives on Organizational Effectiveness,* Goodman, P.S. and Pennings, J.M. (eds.). San Francisco: Jossey-Bass, Inc., Pubs.
6. Jobson, J.D. and Schneck, R. (1982). Constituent view of organizational effectiveness: Evidence from police organizations. *Academy of Management Journal,* 25(1), 25–46.
7. Milton, D. (1988). Challenges of quality assurance program evaluation in a practice setting. *J Nurs Qual Assur,* 2(4), 25–34.
8. Connolly, T., Conlon, E.J., and Deutsch, S.J. (1980). Organizational effectiveness: A multiple-constituency approach. *Academy of Management Review,* 5(2), 211–217.
9. Olsen, M.E. (1968). *The Process of Social Organization.* New York: Holt, Rinehart and Winston.
10. Fawcett, J. (1989). *Analysis and Evaluation of Conceptual Models of Nursing* (2nd Edition). Philadelphia: F.A. Davis and Co.
11. Boulding, K. (1956). *General Systems Theory.* Management Sciences.
12. Hall, A.D. and Fagen, R.E. (1956). Definition of system. In *Systems Engineering.* New York: Bell Telephone Laboratories.
13. Brett, J.L.L. and Tonges, M.C. (1990). Restructured patient care delivery: Evaluation of the ProAct Model. *Nurs Econ,* 8(1), 36–44.
14. Etzioni, A. (1964). *Modern Organizations.* Englewood Cliffs, NJ: Prentice-Hall, Inc.
15. Hinshaw, A.S., Smeltzer, C.H., and Atwood, J.R. (1987). Innovative retention strategies for nursing staff. *JONA,* 17(6), 8–16.
16. Martin, T.N. and Hunt, J.G. (1980). Social influences and intent to leave: A path analytical process model. *Personal Psychology,* 33, 505–528.
17. Pooyan, A., Eberhardt, B.J., and Szigeti, E. (1990). Work-related variables and turnover intention among registered nurses. *Nursing and Health Care,* 11(5), 255–258.

18. Slavitt, D.B., Stamps, P.L., Piedmont, E.B., and Haase, A.B. (1978). Nurses' satisfaction with their work situation. *Nursing Research,* 27(2), 114.
19. Hinshaw, A.S., Smeltzer, C.H., and Atwood, J.R., op cit.
20. Donabedian, A. (1980). *The Definition of Quality and Approaches to Its Assessment.* Vol. 1. Ann Arbor, MI: Health Administration Press.
21. Formella, N.M. and Schroeder, P.S. (1984). The unit-based system. In *Nursing Quality Assurance: A Unit-Based Approach.* Schroeder and Maibusch (eds.). Gaithersburg, MD: Aspen Publishers, Inc.
22. Smeltzer, C.H. (1983). Organizing the search for excellence. *Nursing Management,* 14(6), 19–21.
23. Corcoran, N.M., Meyer, L.A., and Magliano, B.L. (1990). Retention: The key to the 21st century for health care institutions. *Nurs Admin Q,* 14(4), 23–31.
24. Perlman, D. and Takacs, G.J. (1990). The ten stages of change. *Nursing Management,* 21(4), 33–38.
25. Drucker, P.B. (1990). *Managing the Nonprofit Organization: Principles and Practices.* New York: Harper Collins.
26. Malloch, K.S., Milton, D.A., and Jobes, M. (1990). A model for differentiated practice. *JONA,* 20(2), 20–25.

CHAPTER 9

The Evaluation of New Nursing Structures in Single or Multifacility Systems

Doris Milton

In recent years there has been an exponential increase in the number and complexity of major delivery system redesign projects in single and multifacility organizations. Examples of such projects include case management and/or managed care, differentiated RN practice, and use of assistive personnel. This chapter discusses ways in which the structural, process, and outcome issues involved in change of this type can be evaluated.

The information presented in this chapter can be used by any facility contemplating the implementation of new nursing structures and by a facility at any point in the change process concerned with methods of summative or formative evaluation. Special mention will be made of the concerns that arise when a redesign is planned in one or more facilities within multifacility systems.

THE INTERRELATIONSHIP OF STRUCTURAL, PROCESS, AND OUTCOME COMPONENTS

Planning, implementing, and evaluating redesign of nursing or patient care delivery systems rely on structural, process, and outcome components. Each of the components has an influence on the others.

Before beginning any redesign, concerns related to evaluation of each of the components should be addressed.

STRUCTURAL COMPONENTS

Type of Redesign

The first concern is evaluation of the type of redesign that will achieve the desired goal or goals. The initial aspect of what type of redesign is planned focuses on whether the change desired is a change in how nursing is practiced, such as differentiated RN practice, a change in the way nursing care is delivered, such as primary nursing; a change in the way patient/family care is provided, such as case management; decentralized multidisciplinary teams; use of assistive personnel; or a change in the governance structure of nursing or the hospital, such as shared or collaborative governance. A redesign can include just one of these changes or a combination of one or more of these structural types.

When one or more structural redesigns are chosen, it is important for all who are involved to achieve consensus on exactly what this structure will look like. If the structural change is being implemented in different patient care areas or on several units, the commonalities that must be present and the differences that are possible need to be addressed. For example, if case management is the type of redesign being implemented, the planning team may decide that a process of monitoring and tracking patient progress toward critical pathway goals on each unit needs to be in place.

However, differences may exist among units regarding whether that process will be used for all patients or only high risk or high volume patients, only patients admitted by selected physicians, for the patient length of stay or the entire illness episode, or only be coordinated by RNs who are employed full time. In this way, everyone will know what is meant by case management at that facility. It will also be easy to evaluate whether or not, and when, case management has been implemented.

Decisions concerning the type of restructuring are very difficult and time consuming, since redesign is not the reshuffling of the same old pieces.[1] Indeed, when redesigning staff or management roles, Vestal (1989) recommends the building of the role based upon what currently exists.[2]

Purpose of the Redesign

In order to decide whether one component or a combination of components are needed in a redesign, the planning team clearly identifies the purposes of the redesign. What are the reasons for redesign? What objectives will be achieved by a redesign? Examples of common purposes for redesign include improved continuity of patient/family care, increased nurse satisfaction, reduced or more efficient resource utilization by patients and their families, more efficient use of personnel, standardization of patient outcomes, a flatter organizational structure, streamlined management teams, development of collaborative practice, and increased patient/family satisfaction with care and preparation for discharge.

The planning team then considers whether the component or combination of components selected for redesign will achieve their objectives. Each component or combination of components may be very worthwhile, but may not change what needs to be changed at that facility. It is important to think about what needs to be altered so that the objectives for the redesign will be met. For example, changes may not need to be made in the governance structure, if nurses are very satisfied with the degree of control they feel they have over their practice and their work environment. On the other hand, if increasing control over nursing practice and the work environment is one of the major objectives of the redesign, then a redesign that does not include a governance component cannot be expected to be successful.

CONGRUENCE OF REDESIGN WITH ORGANIZATIONAL AND UNIT CULTURE

Many redesigns have problems in the implementation phase and some are never fully implemented because of incongruities between the assumptions underlying the redesign and the assumptions held by the unit and/or organizational culture. The culture of a unit or organization may share values and views that conflict with critical assumptions upon which a redesign is based. Also, a new nursing structure may "work" on one unit and not on another solely due to culture conflicts.

Examples of values and assumptions warranting examination and clarification when considering the type of redesign to be used include: the nature of nursing and how its knowledge and skill base differs from that of other disciplines; differences in nursing knowledge and skills created by varied educational preparations and experiential learning; and the roles of staff nurses, managers, and administrators. Values and assumptions that are part of the unit and organizational cultural structure but can influence the process of redesign implementation include: the degree of trust that can be placed in others with roles different than one's own; how much and what can be communicated to whom and when; how much accountability for implementing change is desired; and how much change is tolerated at one time.

Often, different strategies for redesign need to be used if the change that is contemplated is in conflict with, rather than congruent with, the unit or organizational culture. We frequently blame the redesign when it cannot be implemented: "Differentiated practice was just not appropriate for our facility." It may not be the fault of the structure of the redesign, but rather that the redesign was in conflict with the assumptions held by key leaders within the organization.

ROLES OF ASSISTIVE PERSONNEL

Whether a redesign focuses on a change in nursing roles or a change in the method of nursing or patient care delivery, much discussion takes place regarding the roles and potential roles of assistive personnel or nurse extenders. Most redesigns focus on an increased utilization of the knowledge and skill base of RNs. The process of finding ways to use RNs more efficiently quite naturally leaves an extensive list of tasks that RNs are performing that do not require a registered nursing knowledge and skill base.

The recent literature is replete with articles that criticize the ways in which RNs' time is used. Also common in the literature are articles describing positions that have been developed to assist RNs or to extend their capabilities. Positions such as unit assistants, unit hostesses, and nursing assistants, technicians, and aides have been developed or existing positions have been increased or redesigned.

There are many nurses working in facilities today who are concerned about this trend and feel that it may be another cycle. That is, in the past, nursing had times when there were a number of these type of positions. Then the trend switched to an all RN staff, and now we are "going back" to the "way it was before." There is, however, a major philosophical difference in the current trend from the use of these personnel in prior cycles. What appears to be occurring now is a focus on the tasks that need to be performed and an isolation of those that require a RN knowledge and skill base. Those tasks are then retained by RNs. The remaining tasks are grouped and personnel with the minimal base needed to perform those functions are hired. This is different from previous cycles in that these personnel are not given patient assignments, but rather task assignments.

This difference appears to be based on what Prescott (1989) describes as a conceptual reframing of the nursing shortage. That is, there may not actually be a shortage of nurses, but rather a shortage of professional nursing care being provided. This shortage of professional nursing care occurs when nurses are too busy performing tasks that do not require their knowledge and skill base.[3] This conceptual reframing may have led also to the recent trend to call these nonprofessional workers "assistive personnel" rather than "nurse extenders." In fact, they are present to help with tasks related to overall patient care. Personnel performing nonprofessional nursing tasks cannot "extend" the nurse since they do not have a nursing knowledge and skill base and, therefore, are not practicing nursing.

This identification and grouping of nonprofessional nursing tasks in order to identify the most appropriate care provider can assist also in differentiation of nursing functions. Once nursing and non-nursing tasks are isolated, it becomes clear that nursing functions can be grouped as well. For example, Primm (1986) has differentiated at least two RN roles, based on formal educational preparation.[4] Many hospitals have used Primm's work or similar models to develop either pure or transitional models of RN role differentiation.

IDENTIFICATION OF REDESIGN RESOURCES

An important structural element to evaluate due to its influence on redesign is that of resources. Depending on the type of redesign, differing types of resources may be needed. If some resources are not available within the facility or on a consultant basis, a different type of redesign or a phasing in of the desired redesign may be needed. Resources needed will, of course, be most dependent upon the discrepancy between the design that is wanted and where the facility is in relation to the new design. Regardless of the type of redesign, financial resources are needed for support of meeting time, copying of materials, and data collection and analysis. Also, the costs associated with the opportunities that will be lost during the redesign process need to be considered.

The most critical resources are "people" resources. Managers expert in both the content of the change and the process of facilitating that type of change are essential. The continual shaping of a different mind set or culture requires managers who know what type of redesign is planned. They also need to be willing to facilitate the development of others while, in many cases, their own role is changing simultaneously. Personnel who are expert in staff development can provide the formal and informal programs needed for role change and enhancement. An expert is also needed in outcome measurement, as well as data collection and analysis strategies, in order to monitor the ongoing results of redesign.

Most who have experience with restructuring projects also recommend that a project director or coordinator of the planning team be named. Someone with the responsibility of monitoring progress in the redesign effort is needed. In today's busy environment, it is easy to have efforts toward a redesign diverted due to quite benign occurrences. For example, people can make "minor adjustments" in the plan for their unit. These adjustments may lead that unit down a path that is philosophically different than that of the rest of the organization. Also, when change occurs slowly, it is difficult to realize that certain aspects of the redesign have occurred. Elements of redesign become incorporated into "this is how we operate" and the change is no longer identified as "a change." One person with the responsibility to track such happenings can monitor the progress toward redesign most effectively.

The other major resource needed is time. Staff and manager time means increased fiscal resources during the change. Overcommunication between and among those involved in the redesign is not possible. Adequate communication means much time, depending on the type of redesign, is needed for meetings and one-to-one discussions. It is easier to identify staff time needed, because in many cases, it is additional time, or coverage is needed for patient care. Manager time is not as easily isolated, since redesign efforts are usually "incorporated" into their current positions. Managers need a resource, too, to assist them in prioritizing among all of the important projects on which they are working. They also need a sounding board for times when managers are frustrated with change efforts, or are unsure what, if anything, is changing. Managers need a resource whom they can trust to give them accurate feedback and encouragement.

PROCESS

The processes that need to be in place before change is planned or implemented are dependent upon many factors. The type and extent of the redesign being considered, the purpose of the redesign, the resources available, and the unit or organizational culture influence the processes needed. Especially important elements of the culture that affect the processes are the usual ways that change is perceived and accomplished at a facility. The customary methods may work, but because a redesign may be more complex than any prior change, new patterns may need to be developed.

PREPARING FOR THE IMPLEMENTATION OF NEW NURSING STRUCTURES

Culture

Assessment of the structure of a unit and/or organizational culture influences factors to be evaluated to determine the effect of that culture on the change process. If the usual norm is that change is not tolerated well, especially if that change is major, then strategies to prepare the unit or organization for change are needed. For example, the initiation of planned minor changes that have a high likelihood of success may decrease the threat of major change. Much of the change process depends upon the discrepancy between what the extent of the new nursing structure calls for and where the unit or organization actually is at the start of planning. An accurate evaluation of that discrepancy helps to identify techniques that range from total framework implementation to phasing in a series of gradual changes. Often, the total redesign can be implemented on pilot units first. After any minor issues are worked out, the redesign can then be implemented throughout the organization. Most experts suggest, however, that piloting of a redesign occurs on at least two units. If the change is piloted on only one unit, it is difficult to evaluate whether the problems that occur during the pilot phase are due to the change itself or to any one of a complex of factors.

Evaluation of the unit and organizational culture can also help to identify ways in which change is better accepted on a unit or in the organization. On one unit, change is best accepted if presented to all staff simultaneously, while on another, key staff nurses on the evening shift need to be informed before the change is presented at a total staff meeting.

THE PLANNING GROUP

Evaluation of the organizational culture provides assistance in deciding who will be part of the beginning planning team. Most organizations find that either of two approaches works best. The beginning brainstorming and preliminary redesign outline can be developed by a group of administrators and nurse managers, with others in key staff positions incorporated, to complete the redesign structure and process. Some organizations find that having key people from a variety of line and staff positions involved from the beginning is more consonant with their culture. Additionally, depending on the scope of redesign and the organizational culture, a consultant from outside of the organization may facilitate the redesign process in the initial development stages. Monthly meetings are suggested for the planning group throughout the redesign process.

Regardless of which approach to forming a planning group is chosen, a project director needs to coordinate, facilitate, and monitor the redesign process. Selection of a project director is an important one since the person needs expertise in "nondirecting," yet must be able to expedite the process of change. The project director role is one of expediting the development of the type of design, the purpose and objectives of the design, as well as monitoring project progress and communication flow.

At the initial meetings of the planning group, a process for monitoring the progress of implementation needs to be decided. A method of tracking issues that are discussed, but not resolved, at prior meetings is essential. It is frustrating to examine prior meeting minutes to determine how an issue was resolved, only to find that the issue was discussed, but a decision was not reached. Many decisions needing resolution are tabled until the next meeting, but never appear on any subsequent agenda. Also, ways in which conflicts are handled and resolved, both at meetings and the time in between meetings, need to be decided before a conflict occurs.

STAFF AND MANAGER DEVELOPMENT

Continual development, both in the preparation and implementation stages, of staff and management is critical for the role change that occurs in both during redesign. In order to be committed participants, all involved need to know exactly what redesign is planned and the processes that will be used. The more complex the change, the more time it takes to explain it and for all to truly understand the change.[5] Often, a lack of understanding creates a misinterpretation of the change and its implications. Resistance to change is often disguised misunderstanding.

Accurate information and preparation of all involved are key to commitment. Most people do not mind a role change, as long as their fear of not being able to perform in the new role is removed. It is wiser to err on the side of "overinforming" then to give the impression that some information is being withheld. If, for example, the new structure will be piloted on two units, it is still best to provide information to the other units who will not be involved initially. Those who work in departments other than nursing also need a minimum of an overview of the redesign. Any change in nursing, structure or process, influences the activities of all disciplines.

RECORDING

Information that is central to the progress of the redesign and events that seem peripheral to the entire process are important to document. Meeting minutes chronicle progress and provide a way of finding consensus decisions easily. Documentation of brainstorming sessions are helpful when changes in direction are needed. The role of recorder is crucial; accurate documentation of discussions is irreplaceable. Recording of events that occur during planning and implementation are helpful in understanding the reasons for progress or the lack thereof. Monthly documentation of incidents that affect redesign progress can assist in evaluation. Occurrences such as manager changes, policy shifts, hires and terminations, and units opening or closing influence progress, but the exact timing of such events is difficult to recall in retrospect.

COMMUNICATION

Evaluation of the current process for communicating change and the extent to which that process will be effective during a major redesign is a critical consideration. Records of planning discussions, including brainstorming sessions, are helpful to review after a meeting and may even stimulate other ideas or suggestions. Minutes of planning and implementation meetings and feedback that occurred may be important to those who attended the meeting as well as to others not at the meeting. A distribution and posting list for minutes, and a method of verifying that all on the list are continuing to receive and read them, helps to keep everyone informed. Updates at staff, department, and interdepartmental meetings help to ensure the accuracy of information and build support.

Whatever processes are used, the importance of one-to-one communication cannot be overemphasized. During these interactions, allowing time for feelings, both positive and negative, to be expressed about the change builds the support and trust needed for a smooth implementation course. There are a variety of ways in which staff and managers can participate. Guidelines for the most effective ways of doing so are more likely to be heard during informal communication.

OUTCOME

The outcomes of any restructuring project that requires evaluation are the results of the effort expended. The results of the redesign include the degree of success that was achieved in implementing the desired structure using the planned processes, as well as to what degree the structural and process modifications achieved the purposes for which those changes were created.

Structural and Process Outcomes

Before beginning any redesign, criteria need to be in place so the facility knows the redesign matches the planned structure and that it is in place. Also, the culture of the individual units and the total organization needs to be the one desired. If outcomes are not exactly as planned, examination of the influence of the resources that were used and their impact on the project is indicated. An effective planning group, staff and manager development programs, as well as successful recording and communication processes are outcomes of the redesign.

Result Outcomes

Evaluation of the results of any redesign evolves directly from the initial objectives for the change. The terms "results" or "outcomes" are actually misleading, since data that show the effects of progress are usually collected at baseline and throughout the project, not just at completion.

Data that can help to objectively examine the worth of the new nursing structure are based on the objectives or purposes of the program. The most common groups of data collected are related to nurse, patient, and fiscal outcomes. This is because most objectives of restructuring projects relate to improvement in one or all of these three areas. Data in these domains are used to monitor the redesign progress, make adjustments as necessary, and to examine the effects of any modifications made.

VALIDITY AND RELIABILITY CONCERNS

Measures that provide clear evidence of results, positive or negative, of any redesign, need to be selected prior to other planning efforts. Most hospitals are not oriented to research and program evaluation and may have difficulty initially in dealing with a researcher or evaluator's concerns regarding validity and reliability of any measures used. Many different types of data are collected in hospitals and the initial response of administrators and planning group members is to "use what we already have."

Encouragement is needed to examine the data that do exist to determine whether those data are measuring what the planning group intends to measure, that is, that the data are valid. For example, patient acuity may affect redesign efforts and, therefore, be important data to collect at baseline and throughout the project. The actual index of patient acuity at the hospital, however, may not be sensitive enough to pick up any but major changes in patient acuity status. In that case, the index may not be measuring what it is intended to measure.

Also, the extent to which a measure provides stable and consistent results when used with a specific population, that is, its reliability, influences the confidence one has in the data collected. For example, patient acuity status data can vary depending upon which nurse completed the tool. In that case, even if major changes in patient acuity were noted, one could have little confidence that those data reflected an actual change in patient status.

QUANTITATIVE VERSUS QUALITATIVE APPROACHES

A significant challenge in determining which measures will provide the best evidence of results of redesign is in the selection of the best approach, or combination of approaches, to collecting data under real life circumstances. Quantitative or qualitative approaches can be used or a package of measures that uses both approaches may provide the best data.

Quantitative measurement uses instruments to collect data in certain predetermined response or analysis categories.[6] One common quantitative measure used is a tool that measures nurse work satisfaction. The developers of that measure decided which factors related to work satisfaction are important and are likely to change during implementation of a project. In completing such a measure, nurses respond by indicating the degree to which they are satisfied in relation to each factor.

Qualitative methods of measurement use open-ended questions or observation without any attempt to limit participants' responses or behaviors or to fit the responses or behaviors into predetermined categories.[7] Using this type of approach to measure nurses' work satisfaction, nurses might be asked to respond to a question such as "What factors most influence whether or not you are satisfied with your work and how satisfied are you with those factors?"

There are advantages and disadvantages to using either quantitative or qualitative approaches to measurement. Using a quantitative approach to measuring work satisfaction has the advantage of yielding data concerning how satisfied all nurses are with a few important factors. However, there may be factors other than those measured that influence work satisfaction and perhaps influence satisfaction to a greater extent than those factors measured. Often a mix of both quantitative and qualitative approaches permits the collection of data in predetermined categories as well as allowing for the richness of serendipitous information.

NURSE, PATIENT, AND FISCAL RESULTS

Results of a redesign that need to be measured are directly related to the goals the change is expected to influence. Most redesign projects are expected to show a positive impact on a variety of nurse, patient, and fiscal measures. The desire to improve results in these areas is often the impetus to planning a redesign.

A variety of measures exist to examine nurse data since it is the assumption of most projects that improvement in the work environment for nurses will improve quality of care and financial results. Measures that are frequently used include: work satisfaction,[8] organizational commitment,[9] and retention, stability, and turnover rates.[10]

Patient or quality of care related measures commonly used include: patient/family satisfaction with care, patient complications, length of stay and documentation of adherence to criteria for use of the nursing process, and discharge planning. Satisfaction with care is often measured both during and after discharge. This is because actual patient/family satisfaction with care is affected by the degree to which the patient and family were prepared for care after discharge, as well as the care received during hospitalization.

Incidences of complications, such as falls, nosocomial infections, and medication errors, although routinely collected and easily available, are considered incomplete data. This is because improvements in these indicators do not measure an actual increase in the quality of care, but rather a decrease in negative outcomes. Length of stay data are difficult to use since they are usually available as means and a small number of outliers can skew results. Also, many factors other than redesign are likely to affect length of stay.

Fiscal data are kept by all facilities and, therefore, are easily available. It is hoped that a new nursing structure will maintain or reduce a variety of operating costs, even when those costs are balanced against the costs of redesign. Since personnel costs are the largest budget component, operating costs in that area are often expected to decrease. Results such as decreases in orientation costs, supplemental agency usage, and overall FTEs or costs/FTE are frequently examined. A variety of measures that would indicate increased productivity, such as changes in skill mix or nurse/patient ratios, are also used.

In considering which results to examine, two major factors are critical. One factor is the determination of which results can legitimately be expected to be influenced by a redesign. For example, if increased use of assistive personnel is a structural component of the redesign, then an expectation that numbers of full-time equivalent employees will decrease cannot be expected. The second factor is a concern regarding the validity and reliability of any data that are used. If financial data, such as absenteeism costs, are calculated by several unit managers, then each must use the same method consistently for those calculations.

DATA COLLECTION ISSUES

Once a determination is made of which data are to be collected, plans for data collection times are established. Some data need to be collected monthly, some quarterly, and others on an annual basis. For each result that will be followed over time, it is imperative to establish a baseline. Otherwise, it is difficult to know whether selected results are actual improvements.

Other concerns arise from many facilities' inexperience with long-term projects involving data collection. It is not easy to maintain interest in data collection over the long time period of a redesign project. Many seem enthused at the inception of the project, but after a few months will begin wondering how long this collection of data will continue.

Also, there are many changes that occur over time. For example, the people in positions change, so that the person who understood what data were needed and why has gone and the replacement person may not know that the data are needed. Some data are kept only by a specific person, and when that person goes on vacation, no one else obtains the data. Changes also occur in the ways in which data are kept, or even in the actual data that are kept. For example, a decision may be made to change from a hospital-wide to a focused infection control surveillance method. That decision may eliminate the possibility of obtaining specific information that was being tracked regarding nosocomial infections.

Additionally, operational factors continually interfere with data collection. It is difficult to get upset when essential data are not collected, since the damage is unintentional. Data are needed concerning the effect of a redesign on a busy clinical area, yet it is difficult to make data collection a priority during a hectic period on a unit. Also, research activities are not fully integrated into staff or management roles, and are automatically viewed as having a lesser importance than many other endeavors.

MULTIFACILITY SYSTEM CONCERNS

Facilities that are part of a multifacility system and are contemplating new nursing structures have special concerns that need to be addressed. One facility may be the only system component that is planning a redesign. More commonly, though, several components of a system may be contemplating new nursing structures. In either case, the redesign in any one facility impacts another, whether or not the other facilities appear to be involved.

SINGLE FACILITY REDESIGN

If only one facility in a multifacility system is planning redesign, the major concern of that facility needs to be whether the specific redesign that facility is planning or the idea of redesign itself is incompatible with the overall system culture. The goals of the redesign need to be in concert with those of the organization. Also, it is beneficial if the specific redesign is consistent with the philosophies of the other facilities.

Often, if a redesign is successful in one facility, others in the system will be encouraged to adopt a similar structure. Conflict between facilities can occur if the leaders in each of the facilities disagree on basic tenets of the redesign structure. Communication among facilities throughout the change process is important so that the facilities not directly involved in the change can respond to questions in a supportive manner.

MULTIFACILITY REDESIGN

When more than one facility in a multifacility system is planning new nursing structures, an evaluation of the structural, process, and outcome aspects of the system-wide implications of new nursing structures is critical to the success of both the individual and system efforts.

Open communication among all facilities in the system, even though they may be at varying stages in the redesign process, is helpful to all facilities.

STRUCTURAL CONCERNS

When more than one facility is planning a redesign, the desired goals of each facility may be different. Therefore, a different design may be needed in each facility. A decision needs to be made concerning the variations in redesign that are acceptable. It may be important at an early stage to decide what, if any, commonalities in the type of redesign need to be present throughout the system.

In some instances, differing structural designs, rather than exact replications of one type of design, may even be encouraged. If facilities are similar, the systems may wish to experiment with several types of redesign. Allowable variations in types of redesign are dependent upon the degree of facility independence and the strength of the system culture.

In some instances, conflicts can arise due to a difference between the individual facility culture and the system culture. For example, the individual facility culture may support major change or flattening the administrative structure, but the system culture may not be supportive of either value at that time. Also, units that appear comparable across facilities, such as critical care units, may have differing cultures and staffing mixes. A redesign that may suit one critical care unit may create massive conflict in another.

Critical assumptions that underlie value systems may vary across facilities. In addition to previously discussed views on how much change is tolerated at one time, facilities can have differing views on design components. For example, facilities that do not agree on a definition of professional nursing practice or the roles of assistive personnel will have difficulty achieving consensus on a structural redesign that incorporates differentiated practice.

A comparison between system-wide objectives and individual facility preferences for redesign can help with planning for eventual change. Clarification of differing value systems, organizational cultures, and patient/staffing mixes, if conducted early in the process, can decrease the potential for future conflict. The temptation in any multifacility system is to mandate that all facilities adopt the structural format of an individual facility redesign, when that redesign was successful in one facility. However well intentioned the motive may be, a new structure that is successful in one facility may be difficult to transplant to another facility. Understanding this reality may reduce conflict in the system. Even when an overall redesign model is agreed upon by the leaders in a system, the model will "look different" in each facility.

Different resources may be available in each facility and those resources can impact both the content of the redesign and the speed with which the redesign can be implemented. If facilities in the same system have good working relationships, resources can be shared or pooled so that all facilities benefit. Resources for manager and staff development, project planning and evaluation, and data analysis are most efficiently used when shared among facilities. In some systems, if facilities are planning similar redesigns, a single project coordinator may assist in maintaining the structural integrity of the redesign.

PROCESS CONCERNS

Communication between and among facilities is the single most important process concern in multifacility systems. This becomes especially essential to avoid misinformation communication when redesign efforts are underway. It is critical for each facility to have full information about the structure of the redesign in each facility, the progress that has or has not been made, and the outcomes of the redesign as data become available.

The tendency is for those at each facility to become very familiar with their redesign and emotionally invested in its success. When this occurs, it is easier to disparage the efforts of other facilities. Personnel at each facility wonder aloud why the other facilities are not just automatically adopting the new nursing structure at their facility, since it is obviously the best one. Support of the efforts of each facility by those in other facilities is integral to system success. When adequate information is not available, personnel at each facility speculate on what may be occurring. Rumors begin concerning the money that is or is not being saved or the nurses that are being laid off or hired. Not only are most speculations incorrect, but they can affect the success of all efforts being made within the system.

When several facilities in one system are involved in redesign projects, a natural competitiveness evolves. Although it is important to foster a facility commitment, this competition can be destructive if facilities achieve varying degrees of success. On beginning redesign efforts, a plan needs to be developed to provide support for all of those efforts, not just those that achieve the desired outcomes. This is especially true if the agreement is for facilities to experiment with different structural redesigns.

OUTCOME CONCERNS

When more than one facility in a system is evaluating new nursing structures, it is important to achieve consensus on a common minimum evaluative data set. Each facility may collect additional data if their redesign is for a vastly different purpose, but it is possible to obtain agreement on common nurse, patient, and fiscal outcomes.

If several facilities are interested in improving nurse satisfaction, for example, it is wise to use the instrument that is the most valid, reliable, and sensitive to change in all facilities. If one facility has a specific concern other than what is accepted as part of the minimum outcome data set, those data can be collected and analyzed separately for that facility. For example, if one facility wished to improve physician satisfaction with nursing care, measurement and analysis of data related to that concern can be conducted for that facility.

In multifacility systems it is often assumed that, since they are recording the same data, data definitions are similar. For example, if vacant nurse position data are kept in each facility and a reduction in vacant nurse positions is a desired outcome in several facilities, those data need to be examined to determine if they actually are defined in the same way. What is considered to be a vacant nurse position in one facility may not be considered a vacant position in another. When reporting outcome data, one facility finds it has reduced vacant nurse positions by 25% and another by 50%, yet they may both have actually reduced vacant nurse positions by the same amount. Also, data kept in all facilities may have different degrees of reliability, since they are kept by personnel with varying backgrounds and purposes for data collection.

CONCLUSION

It is hoped that this overview and discussion of real life evaluation of structural, process, and outcome issues is of benefit both to those contemplating redesign in a single facility or multifacility system. In today's rapidly changing health care environment, redesign seems inevitable if we are to maintain our capability for providing cost-effective, quality care for patients and their families. As Barry and Gibbons (1990) recently stated, "Changing circumstances have become so compelling that it is no longer a question of *whether* familiar systems need redesigning, but rather *how soon* and *by what means* a different system will take the place of the existing one."[11]

QUESTIONS

Type of Redesign

1. What type of new structure do we want? Is there one component or a combination of components in our redesign?
2. What commonalities must be present in the structure of our redesign? What individual unit differences are permitted or encouraged? What indicators will we use to identify that our redesign is in place?

Purpose of the Redesign

3. What is the purpose of our redesign? What objectives will we achieve through redesign?
4. What needs are being met by our current structure? What needs are not being met by our current structure?

Congruence with Organizational Culture

5. What are the elements of our organizational culture? What are the elements of the culture on the units that will be involved in the change?
6. What assumptions do we hold about nursing? the practice of nursing? the differentiation of types of nursing knowledge and skills? the role of staff, managers, and administrators? Do we have consensus regarding these assumptions?
7. Is our culture in conflict with the redesign we want? If so, what elements of our culture will need to change? What elements of the redesign may need to change?

Assistive Personnel Roles

8. Have we delineated tasks that do not require the knowledge and skill base of a professional nurse?

9. What assistive personnel are we using and how are we using them? Will that structure need to change in any way?

Redesign Resources

10. What resources do we need to facilitate the redesign planned? Do we have those resources in our facility or are they available to us?
11. Is a project director or coordinator needed? What will that person's role and functions be?

Cultural Assessment

12. Is the organizational culture supportive of the change? Is the unit culture supportive of the change?
13. What is the discrepancy between the structure we want and the structure we now have? Will a total framework implementation or a phasing in of the redesign work best for our facility?
14. What strategies have worked well in the past to facilitate change?

Planning Group

15. Who needs to be a member of the planning group so that the new structure will be accepted by the unit or organization? How often does that initial planning group need to meet?
16. Is there a person within the organization who could serve as a project director?
17. What process will work best for monitoring implementation progress? How will conflicts at meetings and between meetings be resolved?

Staff and Manager Development

18. What are the developmental needs of managers prior to redesign? How do those needs differ from the needs of staff?
19. How will communication about the redesign with other departments be accomplished? Are there established mechanisms that can be used?

Recording

20. What process will work best for recording events or meetings central to the redesign? Who would best serve as recorder?
21. What process will work best for recording events that are peripheral to the redesign? Who would best serve as recorder?

Communication

22. Will any alterations be needed in the usual way that major changes are communicated in our organization?
23. Who needs to receive minutes of redesign meetings? Who is the most appropriate person to provide updates at staff meetings?
24. Is any developmental work needed to improve the one-to-one communication ability of the managers?

Structural and Process Outcomes

25. Is the redesign structure that is in place the one that was planned?
26. Was the planning group able to facilitate the monitor progress?
27. Did the recording process keep staff, managers, the department, and other departments informed?
28. Did the communication processes used provide for accurate and consistent information and feedback?

Result Outcomes

29. How will we know that the redesign has achieved the objectives we had for that change?
30. What data will need to be collected concerning nurse, patient, and/or fiscal outcomes?
31. At what intervals will those data need to be collected? Do we need to obtain any baseline data in those areas for future comparison?

Validity and Reliability Concerns

32. Are there existing measures that we want to use to collect outcome data? Do other measures need to be developed?
33. Are the measures that we want to use valid and reliable? Are they sensitive enough to pick up changes?

Quantitative vs. Qualitative Approaches

34. Do the measures we want to use to measure outcomes use quantitative or qualitative approaches?
35. Will we be able to obtain all of the information we want by using the measures we plan to use?

Nurse, Patient, and Fiscal Results

36. What nurse, patient, and/or fiscal data will we need to collect? How readily available are those data?

37. Are the data we want collected in a consistent fashion throughout the organization? If not, what can we do to increase the consistency of keeping data?

Data Collection Issues

38. What time intervals are planned for data collection and who will be responsible for monitoring that plan? How frequently will reports of data analysis be needed and how will information from those reports be disseminated?
39. What methods will be used to maintain interest in data collection over an extended time period?

NOTES

1. Madden, M.J., and Lawrenz, E. (1990). Work re-design. In Mayer, G.G., Madden, M.J., and Lawrenz, E. (1990). *Patient Care Delivery Models*. Gaithersburg, MD: Aspen Publishers, Inc., pp. 3–12.
2. Vestal, K. (1989). Job design: Process and product. *Nursing Management,* 2(12), 26–29.
3. Prescott, P. (1989). Shortage of professional nursing practice: A reframing of the shortage problem. *Heart and Lung,* 18(5), 436–443.
4. Primm, P. (1986). Entry into practice: Competency statements for BSNs and ADNs. *Nursing Outlook,* May-June, 135–137.
5. Wilson, C. (1989). The challenge of organizational change: Doing less while being more. *Aspen's Advisor for Nurse Executives,* 4(10), 6–7.
6. Patton, M.Q. (1980). *Qualitative Evaluation Methods.* Beverly Hills: Sage.
7. Ibid., p. 24.
8. Stamps, P.L. and Piedmonte, E.B. (1986). *Nurses and work satisfaction: An index for measurement.* Ann Arbor: Health Administration Press Perspectives.
9. Mowday, R.T., Steers, R.M., and Porter, L.W. (1979). The measurement of organizational commitment. *Journal of Vocational Behavior,* 14, 223–247.
10. Prescott, P. (1986). Vacancy, stability and turnover of registered nurses in hospitals. *Research in Nursing and Health,* 9, 51–60.
11. Barry, C.T. & Gibbons, L.K. (1990). DHHS nursing roundtable: Redesigning patient care delivery. *Nursing Management,* 21(9), 64–66.

CHAPTER 10

A Call for Action

As nursing leaders, practicing in an environment fraught with crisis, we have our own moment of history facing us. We have never really been passive bystanders in the history of health care. Following the rich tradition of past healers, our nursing leaders were instrumental in shaping the present health care system.

Today, we must help to solve the problems of a failing system. This means we must engage in the rethinking of our nursing organizations. We must act upon the strategic and central position of nursing within the whole health care system.

Nursing leaders must purposefully engage in restructuring nursing practice and the systems that support it. This work requires a solid understanding of organizational structure, the courage to deal with organizational behavior, and an intense commitment to keep the workplace professional. The chapters of this book have attempted to address all three of these requirements.

The demands for balancing the cost and quality of care will continue to intensify. It must be recognized that nurses are central to the design, the development, and the delivery of patient care services. With this recognition, certain organizations will flourish. Those organizations that survive the changes of the next decade will succeed because of a certain kind of restructuring effort. Restructuring efforts will deliberately increase access to the knowledge and expertise of professional nurses, in the patient care arena of organizational decision making.

The new nursing organization will possess a reduction of emphasis upon hierarchy, an environment of greater autonomy and participation, a de-emphasis upon rules, and a strong reliance upon the trustworthiness and the self-discipline of professional nurses. There will be few restrictions on communication and a commitment to partnerships.

Perhaps we should look upon our work as an "improvisation act" in which we reorder the familiar and the unfamiliar elements of our nursing organization, to fit our rapidly changing environment.[1] Such a perspective stimulates the creative response that is so necessary for survival.

We can no longer hold onto our cherished traditions. Change is all around us. The risks are too great to not seize the moment. Change may be perilous but stagnation is deadly.

There are several risks in *not* changing. All of the potential scenarios spell certain disaster for quality patient care. The conflict and competition between professional groups for resources and recognition within organizations will intensify, as resources shrink. Some professional groups will come out on top and some will tire of the battle. Those who tire of the battle will withdraw from organizational problem solving. Consequently, patient care decision making will be made from the viewpoint of only a few. Some problems will not even be recognized. Nursing, depending upon the strategic actions of today's nursing leaders, will be part of the solution or part of the problem.

Those professional groups with the most power will dominate the work of other groups. If nursing delivery systems do not clearly define and articulate the professional nursing role, then the needs of other groups will determine nurses' scope of practice. If this happens, requirements for patient care will be determined by the needs of predominant groups. Patient needs will not be matched to nursing expertise. Both the patient and the nurse will suffer.

If we do not realign our organizations to meet contemporary demands, we can risk becoming so depressed about our circumstances that we are doomed to failure. In such an environment, no innovation will be considered effective enough to overcome our deficiencies. Nursing organizations will turn inward and lose their perspective about what is really needed for quality patient care.

Some nursing organizations will look for nurse saviors to implement the ideal new structure. These saviors will turn into dictators, over time. Their new ideas will take on the qualities of a religion. It may look to the outsider that the organization has changed. However, it will be fraught with the same obstacles we face today: hierarchy, blocks to innovation, and a lack of control over our own destiny. Comfort with the status quo will result in a standardization of our approaches to patient care, to the neglect of the individual.

Finally, some nursing organizations will try to rise above the politics and the power struggles inherent in any change. There will be an environment of pseudo-harmony, until reality crashes in. These organizations will only be able to react to the changes initiated by others. Some changes will benefit patient care while others will not.

To choose the pathway of change is easy. The process of implementation, however, is deceptively difficult. Change will put the lives of those we lead into considerable flux. We must assure every step of the journey is taken cautiously but deliberately, in recognition of the human experience of change.

The multiplicity of relationships managed during a change can be avenues of growth for all who are involved. Professional development will accompany change under the right conditions. The chapters in this book have described a few of these conditions. Demands for immediate change must be balanced with taking the time to link actual organizational problems with true solutions. Potential solutions will not simply be laid on top of existing structures. Rather, we will take potential solutions and tailor them to our own use. We will look upon project conception, selection, and planning as the central elements of the change process, with actual implementation as the outcomes of this crucial project management work. Thinking through a change must be as important as acting upon it. We will not attempt change without adequate resources. The politics of change will be anticipated, recognized, and dealt with effectively.

History has not required that nursing be locked into any specific environment. Our collective wisdom, intelligence, emotional strength, and resilience enables us to not just accept our future, but to shape it.

NOTE

1. Bateson, M.C. *Composing A Life*. New York: The Atlantic Monthly Press, p. 3.

Index

D

E

J

L

M

Q

R

S

T

U

V

W

About the Author

Cathleen Kruger Wilson, PhD, RN, is the Senior Partner of Specialty Applications, a full-service consulting practice, providing services to nursing organizations and nonprofit service associations. She has a strong background in nursing administration, professional association leadership and the education of nursing administrators.

Wilson has held positions in nursing administration, association management, graduate education, and clinical nursing specialties. She presently holds an adjunct faculty position at the College of Nursing at Arizona State University, where she teaches in the graduate nursing administration tract. Her numerous speaking and publishing activities reflect her strong background in the management of change, development of professional practice environments, and the implementation of quality management programs.

Wilson has received many honors, including Segma Theta Tau's Distinguished Lecturer Award and membership on the editorial board of the *Journal of Nursing Quality Assurance*. She is presently a member of the American Nurses' Association's national taskforce on workplace advocacy. Her educational preparation consists of degrees from Marquette University (PhD), St. Xavier College (MSN), and the College of St. Teresa (BSN).